HOW TO PASS MEDICAL EXAMS

(A Survival Guide for Medical Students and Doctors)

DR MARC BARTON

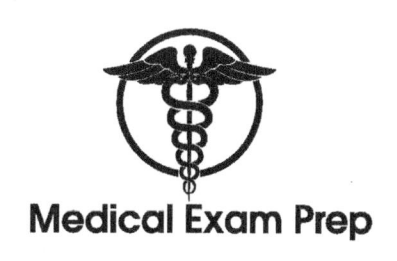

Medical Exam Prep

Notice: The author and publisher disclaim any personal liability, either directly or indirectly, for advice or information presented within this book. Every effort has been made to ensure the accuracy and completeness of information but it should be understood that much of the subject matter contained within this book is not rooted in scientific observation and has come from the authors' own personal experiences. There is considerable variability in the educational requirements of medical students and doctors and some of the recommendations provided may not be universally applicable. No responsibility is assumed for any errors, inaccuracies, omissions, or any false or misleading implication that may arise due to the text.

All rights reserved. Apart from any permitted use under UK copyright law, this publication may only be reproduced, stored or transmitted, in any form, or by any means with prior permission in writing of the publishers.

© Medical Exam Prep Ltd

Dedication

To Mum and Dad, who believed in me when no one else did and made my dream of becoming a doctor a reality with their unconditional support.

To my great friend Nicolas Gregoriades, who gave me the self-belief to start the journey of writing this book.

And last, but not least, to my wonderful wife Clare, who has been by my side since our very first exams at Medical School and has supported me at every step along the way!

Contents

Foreword vii
Introduction ix

PART 1 – GETTING STARTED

1. What is Different About Medical Exams? 2
2. The Basics 5
3. Preparation and Planning 7
4. Reading Material 10
5. Learning Online 13

PART 2 – HOW TO STUDY AND LEARN EFFECTIVELY

6. Types of Learner 22
7. Studying Alone 25
8. Studying in Groups 30
9. Learning in Clinical Practice 34
10. Revision Courses 40
11. Making the Most of Your Memory 43

PART 3 – UNDERSTANDING YOUR EXAM

12. Understanding the Syllabus 50
13. Understanding the Language 52
14. Understanding Acronyms and Abbreviations 63
15. Understanding the Questions 70
16. Understanding OSCEs 86
17. Understanding Vivas 120

PART 4 – THE LITTLE THINGS THAT MAKE A DIFFERENCE

18. Dealing With Stress and Anxiety 126
19. Improving Your Confidence 135
20. The Importance of a Good Nights Sleep 139
21. Food For Thought 145
22. Healthy Body, Healthy Mind 152
23. Meditation and Mindfulness 155

PART 5 – FINAL PREPARATION

24. The Last Few Days 160
25. Re-sits 164
26. On The Day 168

Closing Thoughts 175
About the Author 177

Foreword

If only I knew then what I know now! -- something that most of us have said to ourselves at some point… pointlessly, of course. However, as they say: "it's better to learn from others' mistakes [and others' wisdom] than from your own. They also say that "proper preparation prevents p*ss poor performance!"…. and all of this is true.

All of the above applies as much to exams as to any other aspect of our lives, and if you've chosen a career in medicine then you've condemned yourself to what can, at times, feel like an endless recurring assault of study and exam trauma.

Being a bit of an old-school dinosaur from a bygone era, I received little or no teaching during my training about how best to learn, revise and perform in exams, and probably most of my experience came through trial and error, simply stumbling into what felt most right for me.

The two epiphany moments that I did have that did significantly help shape me were first, failing two out of three of my end of 1st-year exams at medical school (and as a result losing my entire summer holiday to study for the re-sits) and then second, reading an inspirational article in a fitness magazine about sports psychology. It was reading, understanding and following some of the principles of sports psychology and applying this to study and to exams that transformed my approach to the later exams in my medical training, which, despite being the hardest exams ever, I passed first time every time.

Marc Barton was my SHO when I was a registrar, and we have remained friends ever since. I've always seen Marc as a bit of an exam-passing-machine, and he's done more exams and has more letters after his name than almost anyone I know. Marc's also a formidable athlete. The advice that Marc gives in this book comes not just from research but also from extensive personal knowledge and experience, from someone who's been there, who's read the book and who's worn the T-shirt ... and who's now taken the time to share his insight.

If this book had been around when I was younger I'd have bought it, I'd have read it from cover to cover and I've have followed every bit of advice contained within, religiously.

I found this book easy to read and full of common sense and golden nuggets of wisdom, and I hope that you too enjoy it and find value in its messages, and that you have success (and as little pain as possible) in whatever exams you face in your ongoing training in the wonderful world of medicine!

Mr Ian McDermott
MB BS, MS, FRCS(Orth), FFSEM(UK)
Consultant Orthopaedic Surgeon

Ian McDermott is a Consultant Orthopaedic Surgeon specialising in knee surgery. He is the founding member and the Managing Partner of London Sports Orthopaedics, which is one of the country's leading private orthopaedic practices. Ian is also an Honorary Professor Associate in the Brunel University School of Sport & Education. Ian was the youngest ever surgeon in history to be elected as a Council Member and Trustee of the Royal College of Surgeons of England, and he has also sat on the Council of the Faculty of Sport & Exercise Medicine. Ian is currently a Board Member of the Federation of Independent Practitioners Organisations and he is the Private Practice Rep on the Professional Practice Committee of the British Orthopaedic Association. Ian's main clinical interests lie in the fields of knee reconstruction, and he is a leading figure in the area of custom-made knee replacement surgery and in complex soft tissue knee reconstructions, including meniscal transplantation and articular cartilage grafting.

Introduction

I have sat a lot of exams, probably too many. My career in medicine has taken me down various different paths and some of the choices that I have made have been misguided. I have worked in General Medicine, been a GP partner and more recently have worked as a trainee in Emergency Medicine.

Despite my indecision in my career, I have achieved a great deal of success in exams. To date I have passed a Bachelor of Science degree in Physiology, Medical Finals, the MRCP, the MRCGP with distinction and most recently the MCEM examination. I have also sat and passed two diploma exams, the DRCOG and DCH.

I did not pass these exams due to extraordinary intellect or academic prowess, as I possess neither of these. In fact throughout school I consistently struggled with exams and was told on more than one occasion that I didn't have what it takes to become a doctor. I passed these exams because of the methodology with which I approached them. With each exam I sat, I became more and more adept at being able to plan and prepare in such a way that I was able to pass exams that many people much brighter than I had failed. I truly believe that the success that I have had in these exams has been attributable to the precise and methodical approach that I took to preparing for them.

I hope that in this short book I can help you to utilize some of the methods that I have used to pass the exam that you are preparing for. Good luck!

Dr Marc Barton
BSc (Hons), MBBS, MRCP, MRCGP, MCEM, DCH, DRCOG

PART 1

GETTING STARTED

What is Different About Medical Exams?

"There is no end to education. It is not that you read a book, pass an examination, and finish with education. The whole of life, until the moment you die, is a process of learning." – Jiddu Krishnamurti

You are different

By the time you are even in a position to be reading this book you will have prepared for and sat numerous exams. Throughout your schooling you will have prepared for several key examinations to allow you to enter into medical training. If you have already qualified as a doctor and are preparing for a postgraduate exam you will have already 'run the gauntlet' of medical finals.

You may have failed some of these examinations and passed them at a second, or even a third attempt. You may be preparing for your first medical school examinations, your medical finals or perhaps even your final postgraduate exam that is a requirement for your chosen specialty. Each of these exams will be challenging in different ways and will require a vast amount of knowledge and effort to pass.

The process of sitting these exams will have produced a battle-hardened student that has been tested time and time again. You are different to the standard exam candidate because of this.

The exams are different

Unfortunately the exams that you will be sitting are also different. The depth and level of knowledge you will expected to master will get harder at each subsequent step along the path to your final goal. You will be tested on more than just factual recall. To become a doctor requires intelligence and knowledge but also integrity, resolve, technical proficiency, calmness under pressure and many other intangible qualities. Medical schools and colleges attempt to test all of these in the exams they set, in order to ensure that the doctors that they produce will be able to deal with the constant challenges and stresses that medicine presents.

Lifelong learning

By choosing medicine as a career you have chosen a path of lifelong learning. It is highly likely that you have many more exams ahead of you. It is important to be committed to continual self-improvement and knowledge attainment in order to keep up with the ever-changing nature of medical management. The exams that you sit, especially those in the postgraduate setting, will provide you with important tools to equip for you this lifelong learning path.

How can this book help you?

Although you are likely to be an experienced exam candidate already, there are almost certainly still many ways that you can increase your chances of success. Hopefully this short book can help you identify some new methodologies and tricks that will maximize your chances of passing your chosen exam.

Key points to remember:

- ✓ Medical exams test a diverse range of qualities
- ✓ Medics are experienced exam candidates
- ✓ By choosing medicine as a career you have chosen a path of lifelong learning

The Basics

"A journey of a thousand miles begins with a single step." – Lao Tzu

Medical exams are difficult

The first step to passing your examination is to acknowledge that your chosen path is difficult and that a significant amount of hard work is going to be required. There are no short cuts and these exams are a marathon not a sprint. You must be prepared for many difficult months of work in the run up to the exam. If these exams were easy to pass they would not be a suitable means of protecting the standards of the medical profession.

Resistance and persistence

Due to the amount of work that is necessary and the length of time that is likely to be required to prepare for your chosen examination, you are likely to meet resistance at some point during your journey. Resistance is defined as 'the refusal to accept or comply with something'. There will be many times that you just don't feel like sitting down and studying. Your friends may be out at a party or you may have a family gathering that you would like to attend. It may be that you simply find any excuse not to work. Resistance is what is keeping you from sitting down and studying.

Resistance is a common enemy of writers, and author Steven Pressfield has written a book about this called 'The War of Art'. This book is largely about resistance, not only for writers, but also for anyone that is pursuing their dreams and trying to become what they are meant to be. I highly recommend it to all medical students and doctors in training.

Overcoming this resistance is going to be fundamental to your exam success. The exams are hard work, frustrating and in the case of postgraduate exams, expensive. The key to overcoming this resistance is persistence. Persistence is defined as 'the fact of continuing in an opinion or course of action in spite of difficulty or opposition'. This is what will keep you in front of the books on that Friday night when your friends are at that party or while your loved ones are at the family gathering.

Remember why you are studying

Obviously your final goal is to pass your exam but it is important not to forget that you are also trying to become the best doctor that you can. You entered into medical school not to become an exam-passing machine but to become part of a noble vocation. You more than likely love the subjects that you are studying, and the exams are a tried and tested means of providing you with the skills that you will need when you are in the real world seeing and treating patients with real-life problems. If you love the subject you are studying and enjoy the process of learning about it, the exam preparation will become much more rewarding and your chances of success will increase considerably.

Key points to remember:

- ✓ Medical exams are difficult but passable
- ✓ You are likely to experience resistance at some point
- ✓ Persistence is the key to overcoming resistance
- ✓ Remember why you are studying!

Preparation and Planning

"Success depends upon previous preparation, and without such preparation there is sure to be failure." – Confucius

Know your exam

Each medical exam has its own unique style and content. Medical finals vary between medical schools and postgraduate exams vary between colleges. The MRCGP examination is very different to the MCEM examination, which is very different to the MRCS examination and the FRCA examination. Before your start preparing for the medical exam you are sitting it is vitally important that you know your exam.

Try to get hold of a copy of the exam syllabus, either from your medical school or directly from the college setting your postgraduate exam. This syllabus should be the centrepiece of your exam preparation and may well be the most important single document that you read.

Knowing and understanding your exam syllabus can save you countless wasted hours reading irrelevant topics that won't come up in the exam.

Speak to your peers

You almost certainly will know someone that has already passed the exam you are sitting. It may be a friend in the year above you at medical school or a doctor that you work with. They will have been through the process you are embarking upon already and will be able to help you enormously. Ask about the format of the examination, topics that have come up in previous exams and for any tips that they might have.

If possible, try to find someone else that is sitting the exam to prepare with also. Two heads are definitely better than one when it comes to exam preparation. Everyone approaches exams slightly differently and having a study partner can help in numerous ways. I can clearly recall having a concept that I had been struggling to understand for weeks being explained to me in a matter of minutes by a study partner that simply had a different approach to the problem.

Start early and plan ahead

Medical exams take months, not weeks, to prepare for properly. I have witnessed many friends fail exams solely due to leaving insufficient time to prepare. Most of these exams will require 6 months of tapered revision and some even longer. Starting your revision early will prevent panic in the later stages and allow plenty of time to work through the syllabus and spot problem areas that will need more work.

Planning ahead is even more important once you have qualified and are actually working as a doctor. Not only will you have to contend with shift patterns, long hours and tiredness but you will also be older and be more likely to have family commitments. It is vital that revision courses and study leave are booked far in advance. Try to free up the week before the exam from work and other distractions so that you can properly focus in the vital final stages of your preparation.

The law of diminishing returns

The law of diminishing returns states that 'in all productive processes, adding more of one factor, while holding all others constant, will at some point yield lower incremental returns'. This concept is particularly important when preparing for exams. There is little point in continuously focusing on a topic that you enjoy and already know well at the expense of other areas you are less knowledgeable about. This is a common trap to fall into and I have been guilty of it at times. Your time is much better spent getting to grips with the topics that you don't enjoy or struggle to understand.

Preparation and planning 'do's and don'ts'

Do:

- ✓ Read the syllabus for the exam your are sitting
- ✓ Speak to others that have sat the exam
- ✓ Plan ahead and start revising early
- ✓ Book your study leave far in advance

Don't:

- ✗ Waste time reading topics that are not in the syllabus
- ✗ Prepare in isolation
- ✗ Leave your revision to the last minute
- ✗ Keep reading topics that you already know

Reading Material

"The more that you read, the more things you will know. The more that you learn, the more places you'll go" – Dr Seuss

Textbooks

They may be old fashioned but there is still much value to be gained from reading the right textbook. It is very important to ensure that the text you are reading is valid for the exam you are sitting. It is worth checking with your medical school or postgraduate college to see if they have a recommended reading list, as questions are often set from these texts. Recommended textbooks can sometimes be lengthy and very detailed and are often best used as a reference source as opposed to a book that should be read from cover to cover before the exam.

There are often also revision books available that are designed to be an all purpose text for a particular exam. It is worth asking friends and colleagues that have already sat the exam which book they used. Another good place to look for a choice of textbook is Amazon, where readers have often impartially reviewed books; these reviews make it much easier to make an informed decision about the textbook you choose to study from.

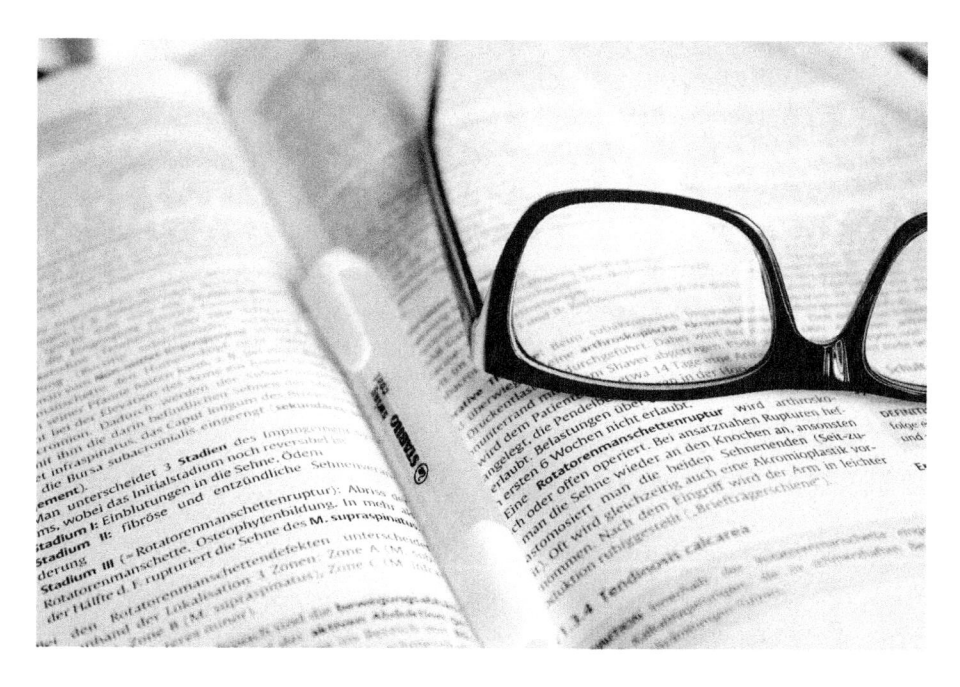

Textbooks may be a little old fashioned but there is still a great deal of value to be gained from reading them.

Alternative texts

There are also some interesting types of alternative texts that are designed to make learning more enjoyable. One particular text that I would recommend to candidates that are sitting the FRCA or any exam that requires a good working knowledge of pharmacology and physiology is 'Gerry's Real World Guide to Pharmacokinetics & Other Things' which is written by Gerald Woerlee. This book manages to teach the basic elements of pharmacokinetics of anaesthetic drugs and some basic physiology by following the conversations of a grumpy senior anaesthetist and a junior anaesthetic resident that is learning the trade. It is genuinely fun to read and this sort of text can help to revitalize the learning process when exam preparation is becoming tedious and difficult.

Practice question books

A large part of your exam preparation should be spent doing practice questions. There are many books available that have practice questions for medical exams. Look for a book that has questions that are similar to those that you will encounter in your exam and that also has detailed explanations accompanying the questions. This type of 'question spotting' can help to point you towards types of topics that are commonly encountered in the exam and also acclimatize you to the style of question that you are likely to encounter. It is a well-accepted fact that students that are familiar with the question style and have practiced these questions do better in the exams that they sit.

Reading material 'do's and don'ts'

Do:

- ✓ Check for a recommended reading list
- ✓ Choose your textbooks carefully
- ✓ Do as many practice questions as possible

Don't:

- X Attempt to read reference texts from cover to cover
- X Use a textbook that isn't relevant for your exam

Learning Online

"When I went to medical school, the term 'digital' applied only to rectal exams." – Eric Topol

An embarrassment of riches

I can clearly remember a time when I had to catch a bus to go to the medical school library to find the resources that I needed to prepare successfully. Things have changed dramatically since then and there are so many different types of learning materials available online that it can be difficult to know what to use and when.

Welcome to the digital age

The advent of the Internet has undoubtedly made exam preparation easier. There are now numerous online sites available specifically designed to help people to prepare for medical exams. Medical schools and colleges often have online lecture material available and there are several good online sites that have practice questions available, an example being www.medicalexamprep.co.uk.

Unfortunately, not everything that you read on the Internet is true, and some information can be poorly presented and difficult to read. Try to look for well-established Internet resources that have input by qualified professionals with training and experience in the field you are studying. It is wise to check the sources of any information that you find and read any references that are listed.

Google Search

Google search is currently the most used web search engine on the World Wide Web and handles more than three billion searches every day. It is a great place to start when researching topics for your exam revision.

It also has numerous search functions that you might find useful during your exam preparation. Here are five that I have personally found particularly helpful:

1. Searching content from a specific website

This can be done using the 'site:' command. For example if you wanted to search for the term 'recent advances in endocrinology' on the New England Journal of Medicine website you could do so by entering: recent advances in endocrinology site:www.nejm.org. Below you can see an example of the sort of results you might expect:

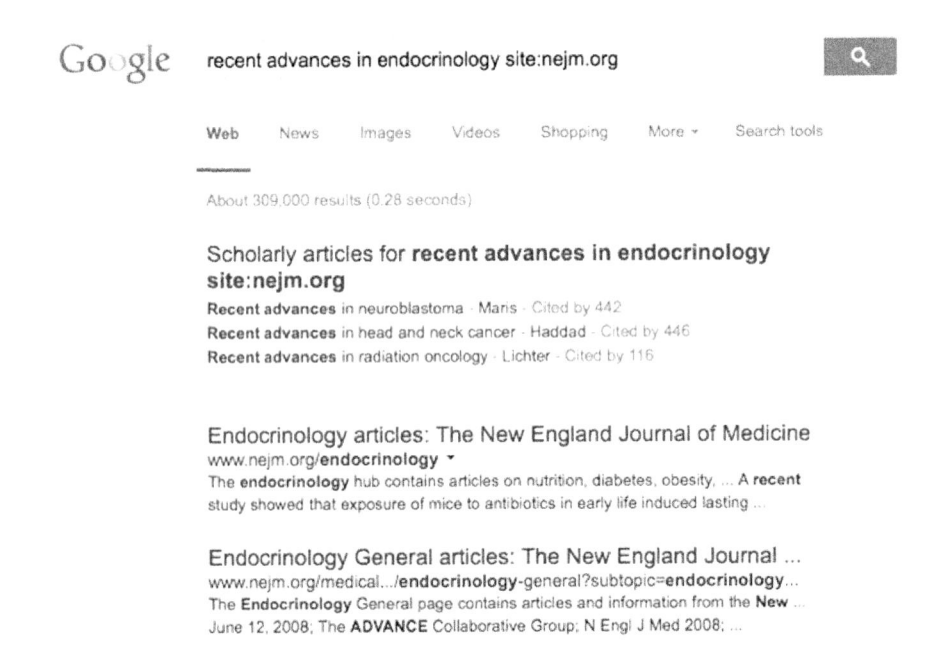

2. Finding definitions

If you are unsure about a word's meaning you can check the definition using the 'define:' command. For example if you wanted to check the meaning of the word 'pneumoconiosis' you could do so by entering define:pneumoconiosis. The definition will then be presented as shown below:

pneumoconiosis
/ˌnjuːmə(ʊ)kəʊnɪˈəʊsɪs/

noun MEDICINE

a disease of the lungs due to inhalation of dust, characterized by inflammation, coughing, and fibrosis.

Translations, word origin, and more definitions

3. Searching with a missing letter or word

If you are attempting to search for a particular word or phrase but cannot remember the exact spelling or wording, Google also has a search function to help with this. By placing an asterix (*) instead of the missing word or letter Google Search will come up with a list of potential alternatives. Here I have forgotten the exact name of an important study on sepsis:

4. Searching for similar websites:

On occasion you may want to look for a website that is similar to another that you are currently using. This can be done using the 'related:' command. For example here I would like to find a website that is similar to the British National Formulary website:

5. Google books:

If you go to http://books.google.com/ you can then search for a book you are looking for either by entering the author's name or the title of the book. This function is particularly useful for checking references from other sources. Here I have searched for Instant Anatomy by Robert H. Whitaker:

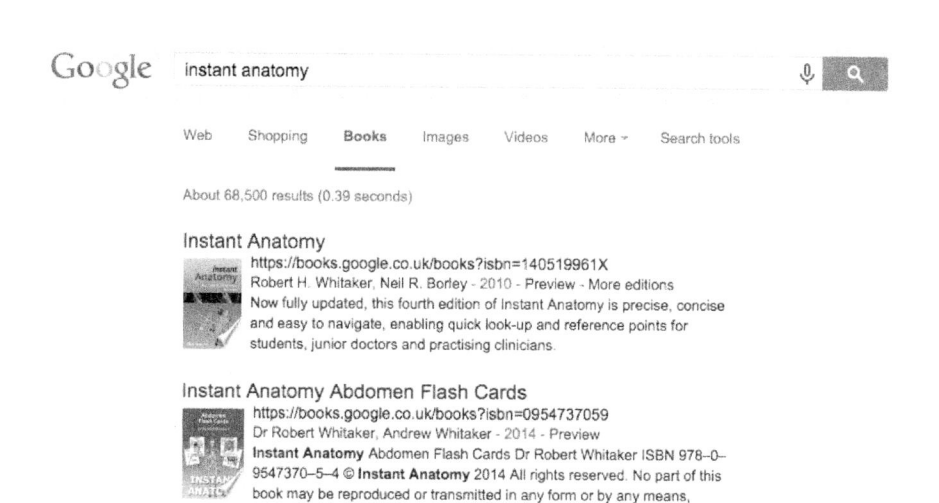

Wikipedia

Wikipedia is a free-access, free content, Internet-based encyclopaedia. It was launched in 2001 and has grown to become the world's largest and most popular general reference work. Almost every medical topic that you can imagine is listed on Wikipedia and it is often the first port of call for students and doctors researching new topics.

Almost anyone can edit any of the articles on Wikipedia and there is no official editorial team. There are at present over 73,000 active editors and over 23,000,000 total accounts. It is a reference source like no other in existence and can be accessed almost anywhere in the world. This has both its merits and disadvantages. The information presented can sometimes be inaccurate and there is no way to check the credentials of the authors. On the other hand, the information is clearly presented and easy to read and incorrect information is generally corrected quickly on most topics.

If you choose to use Wikipedia as a reference tool during your exam revision I would highly recommend cross-referencing any facts that you are not familiar with and inspecting the corresponding reference that is listed at the bottom of the page.

Facebook groups and online forums

Another array of good places to look for advice and support in the run up to an exam are Facebook groups and other online forums and social networking sites. These groups and forums are filled with others such as yourself that are preparing for the same exams. Many people that contribute to the discussions in these groups have already sat the exam and there are sometimes hot topics and questions from previous sittings discussed. They can be a good place to gain insights into the exam you are sitting, get vital tips for your preparation and also to gain support from others in the same situation as yourself.

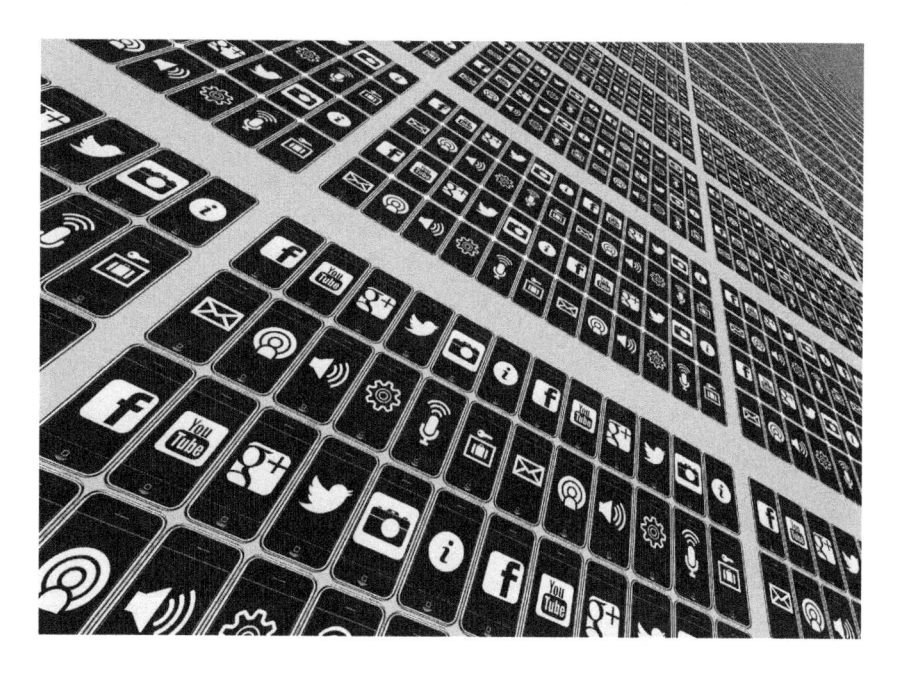

Facebook groups and social networking sites are an excellent place to look for tips and advice

It is worth remembering that medical students and doctors should be careful when posting on social media websites. You should treat colleagues with respect and consideration and protect patients' confidentiality. The UK General Medical Council provides some sound advice on doctors' use of social media, which can be read here: http://www.gmc-uk.org/Doctors_use_of_social_media.pdf_51448306.pdf

Youtube videos

Youtube and online video sites can also be a useful source of information. There are numerous tutorials available as well as mock 'Objective Structured Clinical Examinations' (OSCEs) and videos that guide candidates through technical skills and procedures. These can be particularly useful when preparing for clinical examinations.

A final warning!

The Internet can be absorbing, and at times, extremely distracting. It is very easy to disappear and get lost 'down the rabbit hole' whilst attempting to study. Try not to get distracted by the myriad of diversions that the Internet holds, as before you know it hours will have slipped by with very little gained. I will talk more about how to combat these sorts of distractions in a subsequent chapter.

Learning online 'do's and don'ts'

Do:

- ✓ Look for well-established websites
- ✓ Use an online question bank to practice exam-format questions
- ✓ Utilize the helpful Google Search functions
- ✓ Cross reference unfamiliar facts from Wikipedia and similar sites

Don't:

- ✗ Believe everything you read on the Internet!
- ✗ Forget to respect patient confidentiality when using social networking sites
- ✗ Get distracted by non-relevant online diversions

PART 2

HOW TO STUDY AND LEARN EFFECTIVELY

Types of Learner

"Learning is not attained by chance, it must be sought for with ardour and diligence." – Abigail Adams

Understanding different types of learner

The first step in learning how to study and learn effectively is to understand the different types of learners, and more importantly what type of learner you are. Broadly speaking, there are three types of learner:

1. Visual learners
2. Auditory learners
3. Kinaesthetic learners

Most people learn through a combination of the three learning styles but usually have a clear preference for one. I am predominantly a visual learner.

Here is a short online test, provided by Ashford University, that you can do to work out which type of learner you are: http://www.buzzfeed.com/ashforduniversity/what-type-of-learner-are-you?

Visual learners

If you are a visual learner you will learn best by using primarily visual methods. Visual learners learn most effectively by reading, looking at pictures or watching demonstrations. They tend to have difficulty following spoken directions and can become easily distracted by loud noises and distracting sounds. They are also usually neat and tidy and prefer to study in quiet areas that are free from distractions.

Learning techniques that visual learners find particularly useful include:

- Reading notes from flashcards
- Trying to visualize things you read in your 'minds eye'
- Drawing diagrams to help explain concepts
- Making mind maps
- Colour coding notes
- Writing down key ideas and learning points

Auditory learners

If you are an auditory learner you will learn best by remembering things that you have heard and will find verbal explanations easier to understand than written instructions. Auditory learners learn most effectively hearing, listening and having things explained to them. They often recite things out loud to themselves whilst learning.

Learning techniques that auditory learners find particularly useful include:

- Reciting notes from flashcards
- Reading study notes out loud
- Recording your notes and listening to them
- Having mock exam questions and answers read to you

Kinaesthetic learners

If you are a kinaesthetic learner you will learn best by remembering things through touch and physical movement. Kinaesthetic, or tactile, learners learn most effectively through 'hands-on' experiences. They tend to be active and need frequent breaks in their study. They also tend to gesture with their hands and fidget but be very coordinated and have athletic ability. Sitting still whilst studying can be difficult for kinaesthetic learners.

Learning techniques that kinaesthetic learners find particularly useful include:

- Arranging flashcards into groups to show relationships between ideas
- Learning through 'hands-on' activities
- Acting out scenarios, such as clinical cases
- Solving real-life problems
- Using interactive online learning tools

Key points to remember

- ✓ Understand that there are three main types of learner
- ✓ Do an online test to work out which type of learner you are
- ✓ Try to use the learning techniques that work best for your style
- ✓ Most people learn through a combination of the three learning styles

Studying Alone

"I believed in studying just because I knew education was a privilege. It was the discipline of study, to get into the habit of doing something that you don't want to do" – Wynton Marsalis

Mastering your attention span

Attention span is defined as 'the length of time for which a person is able to concentrate on a particular activity or subject'. Everyone's attention span is different and yours is probably shorter than you think. Most educators agree that the ability to focus attention on a set task is vital to the achievement of any academic goal.

There is no agreed estimate on the average length of the human attention span but for most people it probably lies somewhere between 20 and 40 minutes. Contrary to some people's beliefs, medics are not superhuman and most medics' attention spans will lie in this range also. Understanding this simple fact has helped my exam preparation enormously over the years.

There are numerous online sites where you can take a short test to assess your own attention span. Here is one that you can try yourself, it only takes about 5 minutes, and is a fun way of gaining an insight into your own level of attentiveness: http://testyourself.psychtests.com/testid/3186

I have found that for myself, after a period of about 40 minutes on any single subject, my attention wanes significantly. After a short break of 10 to 20 minutes, however, I have almost re-set to baseline and can spend a similar period of time studying that subject again. I have been able to sustain this method of study from almost dawn until dusk before some exams, with only a couple of longer breaks for meals or exercise. I strongly recommend this approach to personal study and with a little experimentation you should be able to find the perfect balance of study and rest that works for you. Use the short breaks that you take in between your study sessions as a type of reward. Stretch your legs and go for a walk, watch some TV or perhaps even play a computer game.

Set goals and targets

Identifying goals and setting targets is a great way to stay motivated when studying, particularly when studying alone. At the start of your revision I would recommend setting daily and weekly targets and a long-term goal.

For example if preparing for your anatomy exams at the end of the your first year in medical school your long-term goal would be to pass these exams and enter into the second year of medical training. During your revision period a daily target might be to revise the anatomy of the brachial plexus and a weekly target might be to revise the anatomy of the entire upper limb.

Write your targets and long-term goals down and place them somewhere prominent that you will see them on a daily basis, perhaps on your bedroom wall or the fridge door. As you complete each of your targets tick them off so that you can keep track of your achievements and get a feel for what you have left to do.

Avoid distractions

When studying alone try to ensure that you are working in a quiet area that is free of distraction. Try to clear your desk or workspace of clutter once a day and keep all of the books and notes that you will need for your study time close to hand and easy to locate. There is nothing more frustrating than having to search through piles of papers to find that one crucial note or book that you need.

Turn off your home phone, mobile phone, and instant messenger accounts, Twitter, Facebook, TV, radio and any other electronic distraction you can think of. These will interrupt you constantly and it will become almost impossible to concentrate on the task at hand and focus your attention appropriately.

If you are easily distracted by noise, or have to work in a public area, consider wearing headphones or using earplugs to block out any surrounding sound. This will also give people the impression that you cannot hear them and make you less likely to be disturbed.

Unless you absolutely need the Internet I would also disconnect your Wifi and keep away from it. If, however, it is absolutely necessary to use the Internet then you could consider using one of the many available utilities that can be used to block out time-wasting sites for a set period of time. Examples include 'Temptation blocker' and the Firefox Greasemonkey Scripts 'Invisibility Cloak and 'Kiwi Cloak'. Another alternative is 'Time To Go', which will only allow you to surf a site for a certain set period of time.

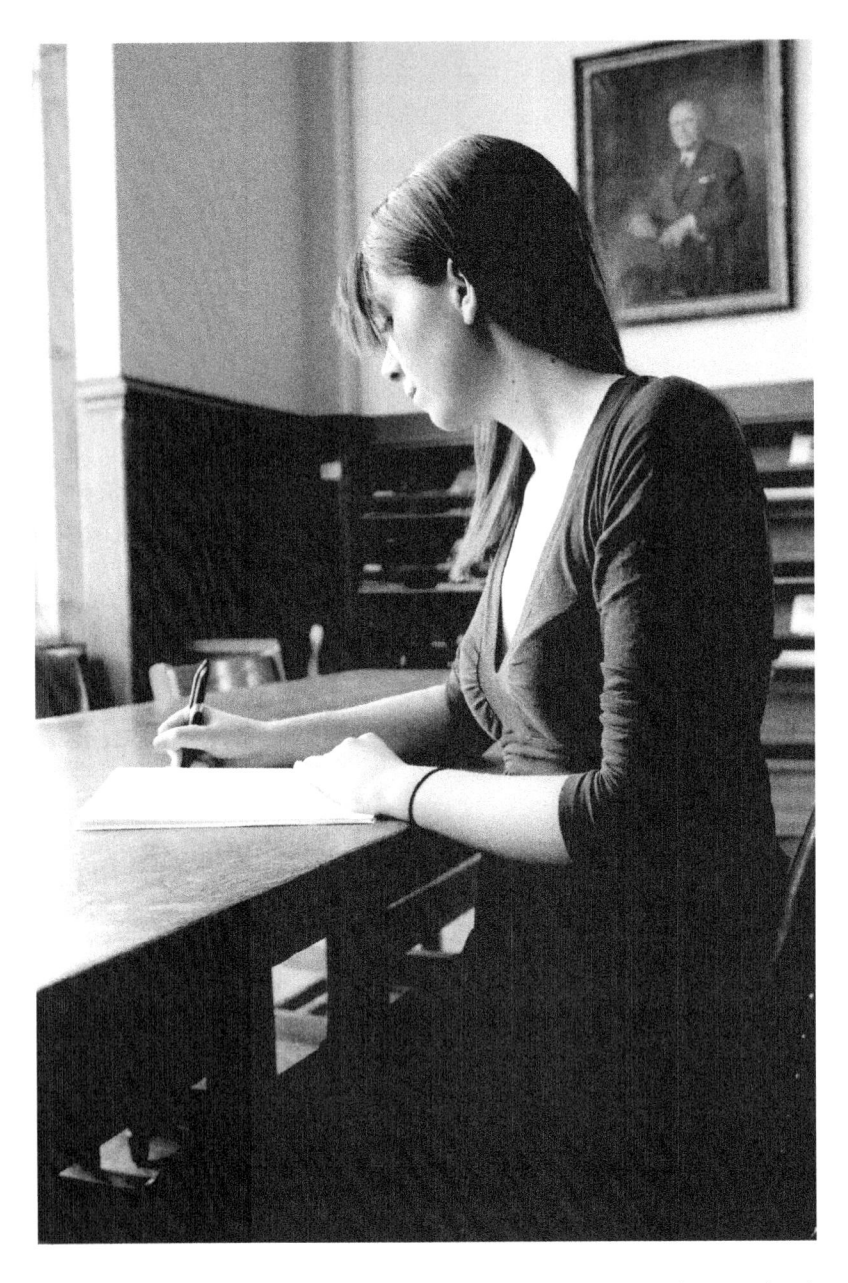

When studying alone try to ensure that you are working in a quiet area that is free of distraction.

Studying alone 'do's and don'ts'

Do:

- ✓ Take regular breaks
- ✓ Set goals and targets for your study
- ✓ Turn off your mobile phone and other electronic devices

Don't:

- ✗ Study for periods of time far longer than your attention span
- ✗ Study in a cluttered workspace
- ✗ Study in noisy areas full of distractions

Studying in Groups

"Alone we can do so little; together we can do so much." – Helen Keller

The benefits of group study

There are a great many benefits to working in groups. Just having others around you to talk to and discuss ideas with can help understanding and stimulate learning. Different members of the group will have different strengths and weaknesses, and by working in a group together you can maximize your individual strengths and minimize each other's weaknesses. Group learning can be dynamic, fast paced and a lot of ground can be covered in a relatively short period of time. It can also be more fun than working alone, and organizing regular group study sessions can provide a welcome relief from the solitude of regular study.

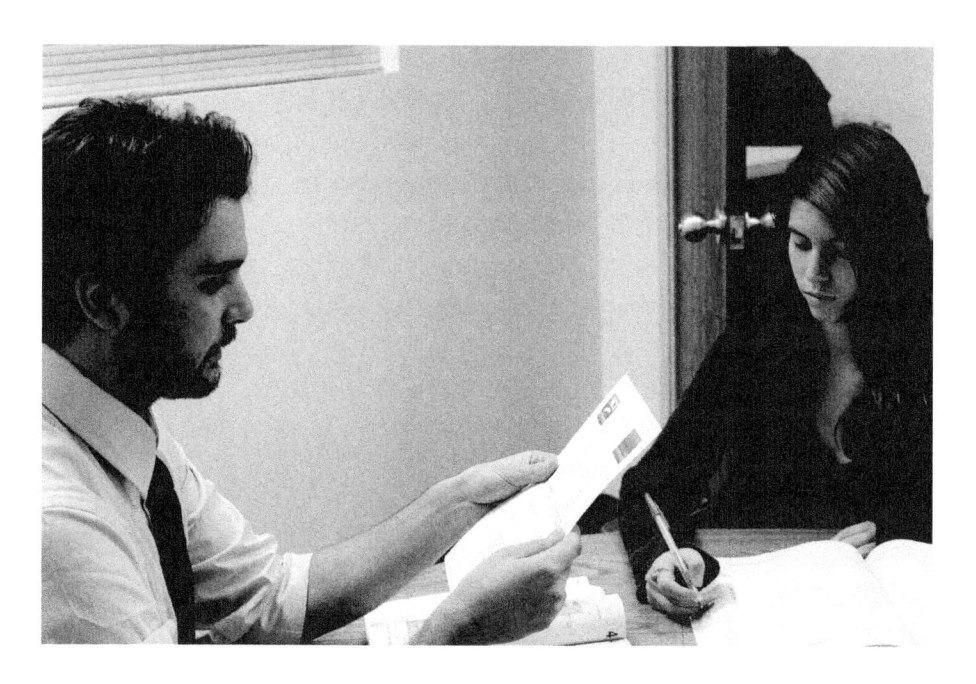

There are a great many benefits to studying in groups and it should form a regular part of your study plan.

Are there problems with group study?

Group study can be an invaluable part of your exam preparation if properly planned and approached in a serious fashion. There is also the potential to waste large chunks of precious time if the group sessions are unplanned and unstructured. I have been part of study groups where the session has disintegrated into a social get together and very little has been gained.

Your study group can be a source of knowledge and understanding but can also be a source of misinformation and misunderstanding. Comments, facts and ideas that are raised in the group setting should be assessed critically and not taken at face value. It is always a good idea to take notes on and further research new and unfamiliar information that is presented in this setting.

Get the numbers right

As with everything else in life, you can have too little or too much of a good thing. A group of two or three people can be productive but that group size is often not large enough to generate a variety of opinions and stimulate the sort of critical debate and discussion that is the ultimate goal of group learning. Likewise, a group of ten or more people is too large for all members to actively participate in and it can be easy for both the agenda and individuals within the group to get lost. In my experience a group size of four or five generally works best and has the best balance.

How to make the most of group study

Try to set an agenda for the study sessions and if possible set rotating topics on a week-by-week basis to ensure that you cover as much of your exam syllabus as possible. Each group member could present a short exam relevant topic that they have researched since the last meeting.

It can be helpful to have an appointed chairperson or group leader. This can help to ensure the smooth running of the sessions and manage the organization of future sessions. If there is no obvious leader then this role can be rotated.

Group study is a great opportunity to discuss past paper questions and debate contentious answers. It can also be helpful to set each other mock questions or mock exams and then discuss how these questions can be best answered.

Try to make the group sessions a regular timetabled event that forms a part of your routine. Meeting once or twice a week for a couple of months before an exam allows a vast amount of ground to be covered.

The timing of the sessions is also important. Anywhere between an hour and three hours can be productive, depending on the content and type of exam that you are preparing for. If you plan on running longer sessions that are two or more hours then make sure you schedule in at least one or two coffee breaks. These act as a reset on your attention span and will allow greater productivity over the course of the session.

Lastly, try to have an open mind and allow yourself to see things from other people's perspective. One of the single greatest benefits of group working is that it can force you to re-evaluate your own ideas and beliefs and integrate new concepts into your practice. For this reason, it is a good idea to work with people that you get on well with and with whom you have an established rapport.

Working in groups 'do's and don'ts'

Do:

- ✓ Appoint a chairperson
- ✓ Set an agenda
- ✓ Make the group sessions a regular timetabled event
- ✓ Discuss past paper questions

Don't:

- ✗ Turn group sessions into social 'get-togethers'
- ✗ Take everything that is said at face value
- ✗ Have too many or too few group members
- ✗ Let group sessions run for too long without breaks

Learning in Clinical Practice

"Isn't it a bit unnerving that doctors call what they do 'practice'?" –
George Carlin

Golden opportunities

Clinical practice holds some of the most valuable learning opportunities that you will be presented with, both as a medical student and as a doctor. These opportunities will continue to present themselves throughout your entire career. You will continually be surrounded by experts in a variety of medical fields, many of whom love to teach and will be delighted to share their knowledge with you. Discussing cases with seniors can be an enlightening, fun and thought provoking way to learn, and knowledge gained in this setting will almost certainly stay with you longer than facts read in a textbook.

One particular study, which looked at medical student activity during clinical attachments, showed that only 40% of the students' time was spent in clinical activity. Another 40% was spent in non-clinical activity such as waiting for teaching and travel, and the final 20% of time was spent on self-directed learning, such as independent study and unsupervised activity with patients. When students were asked to rate the educational value of each activity they overwhelmingly valued time with patients the most and enjoyed self-directed learning the least.

Don't be afraid to ask questions

There is a popular phrase that states 'There is no such thing as a stupid question'. The famous astrophysicist and astronomer Carl Sagan elaborated on this further with the quote "There are naive questions, tedious questions, ill-phrased questions, questions put after inadequate self-criticism. But every question is a cry to understand the world. There is no such thing as a dumb question." No medical student or doctor should ever be afraid to ask a question and it is far, far better to ask a question than to pretend you know something and make a potentially disastrous mistake.

If you don't ask a question that is on your mind then you will have also lost a chance to easily access an answer to that question. It may take hours of research to gain the same insight into a question that could have been answered and explained in a matter of minutes by one of your seniors.

Don't be embarrassed to ask the question in front of other students or colleagues, as they may be too afraid to ask the question themselves and you may in fact be doing them a service.

Learning on the wards

Ward rounds are a great place to learn and prepare for medical exams, both written and clinical. Try to read the notes of the patients that you see and get to know any new admissions by talking to them yourself. Look through the test results of the patients and try to work out the diagnosis yourself. Ask questions about any test results that you don't understand and get a senior to go through important X-ray and CT scan changes. Discuss the patient's management with the team and ask questions about any decisions that you don't fully understand. It is helpful to carry a small reporters style notebook to jot down key points from the ward round that you can read about later.

If you have taken a history from and/or performed an examination of a patient yourself, ask if you can present the patient on the round. This is a great way to get used to presenting and fielding questions in the same sort of way you could expect in clinical exams and OSCEs.

Ward rounds can also be long and tiring. You can spend a great deal of time standing and watching. If you are a student or a junior doctor you can expect to have to fetch and carry items, write notes and do other menial tasks that are required to make these rounds work efficiently. Despite this, these rounds will be very valuable to you and you should try to make the most of them.

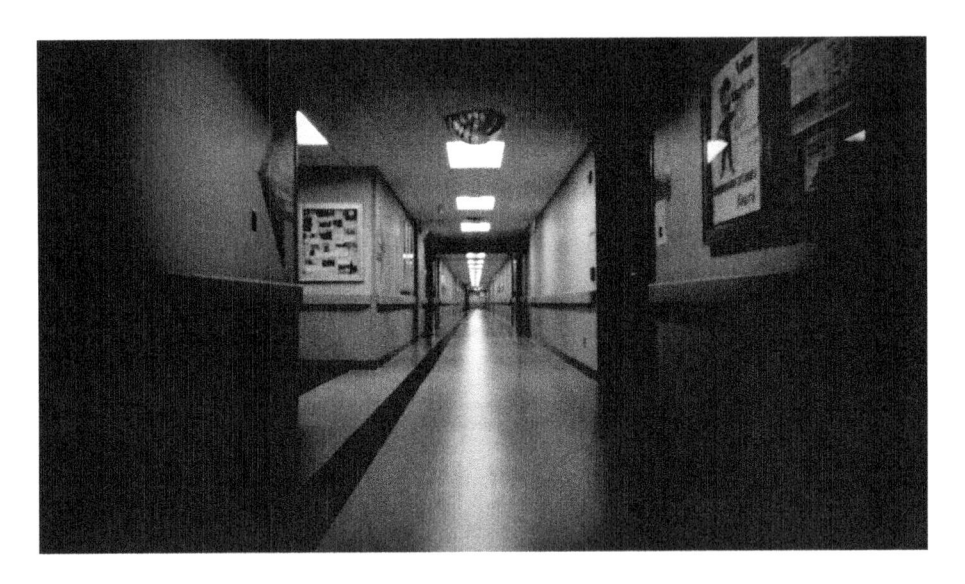

Ward rounds and clinics provide numerous valuable learning opportunities.

Learning in clinics

Learning in the outpatient clinic setting is quite different to learning on a ward round. Clinics can be very busy and time-sensitive, with new patients arriving every 10 to 20 minutes, and opportunities to ask questions and discuss management can be limited by this.

If you are a medical student you are likely to be sitting in with a more senior doctor. Ask if they can brief you about the patient before they come in and if time permits try to read previous clinic notes to familiarize yourself with their medical history. A nice way to learn is to see if an aspect of the consultation can be allocated to you, for example a particular skill or part of the physical examination. This could then be critiqued and discussed after the patient has left the room.

Some clinics that have students and juniors in are allocated more time per patient, but often this is not the case and teaching clinics can sometimes run very late. Under these circumstances try to be patient and understand that the running of the clinic and the patients needs will have to come before your learning experience.

PUNs and DENs

A useful concept to adopt as part of personal learning in the clinical setting is that of PUNs and DENs. PUNs are 'patients' unmet needs' and DENs are 'doctors' educational needs'. These provide a means of exploring educational deficiencies in your own personal time after a consultation with a patient.

PUNs can be explored by asking yourself questions such as "How could I have done better in that consultation?' and 'Did I manage that patient's needs?'. The recognition of a PUN from a particular consultation will then allow you to discover your own personal DEN.

Keep a logbook of the PUNs and DENs that you have discovered and then write reflective notes on them in your own time. You can discuss them with your clinical supervisor or in your study group sessions. You will find that discussing them can provide a very worthwhile learning experience. Make a record in your logbook of how you solved or addressed your educational needs.

Expert patients

Expert patients are defined as 'people living with a long-term health condition who are able to take more control over their health by understanding and managing their conditions, leading to an improved quality of life'. Being an expert patient has numerous advantages for the patient and in addition to being able to contribute to the management of their condition, these patients commonly feel empowered by their knowledge and more in control of their lives.

Expert patients often take great pride in the knowledge they have and are more than willing to help educate medical students and junior doctors to help raise awareness about their illness. These patients frequently have rare conditions and commonly know more about their condition than the physician treating them. Their expertise can present challenges within the consultation, for both the doctor and the patient, but at the same time these patients are a valuable learning resource. Some of the most educational and humbling experiences of my medical career have arisen from managing expert patients.

Try to take the time to sit and chat with these patients about their conditions; not only will it educate you about their particular illness but it will also provide you with valuable insight into what it is like to live with chronic conditions. Another benefit of spending time with expert patients is that they may have experience of being a live patient in a clinical exam or OSCE. They may be able to give you some insiders' tips on things other exam candidates have done particularly well or particularly badly whilst taking a history or examining them.

Learning in clinical practice 'do's and don'ts'

Do:

- ✓ Present patients on ward rounds and in clinics
- ✓ Keep a notebook handy to jot down key learning points
- ✓ Keep a PUNs and DENs logbook

Don't:

- ✗ Be afraid to ask questions
- ✗ Forget to review patient notes and test results before ward rounds
- ✗ Be afraid to talk to expert patients

Revision Courses

"I'd like to share my experiences and the lessons I've learned and hopefully create some amazing, fun courses" – Tiger Woods

Why do a revision course?

I realize that Tiger Woods isn't talking about revision courses for medical exams here, but his quote sums up the value of these courses very nicely. Revision courses aimed at passing a particular exam are often run by doctors that have recently sat the exams themselves and are based on the lessons that they have learned in doing so. The good ones are often fun too.

You can learn many tips and hints about hot topics that keep coming up and exactly what examiners are looking for in the marking schemes. These sorts of insights are invaluable and can make the difference between passing and failing.

Courses exist for both written and clinical exams. Courses aimed at written exams are particularly helpful when essays or short written answers are required. You will often get the chance to sit mock papers under exam conditions, which is a great way to prepare for the exam experience itself. Marking schemes are usually provided and these are particularly helpful. These sorts of courses are also helpful for topics that medics are traditionally less familiar with, such as statistics and critical appraisal.

In my personal opinion, the greatest value of revision courses lies in preparing for clinical exams and OSCEs. These courses essentially become an intensified version of ward-based learning, whereby actual patients can be seen in small groups. You will be able to see far more patients in a single day than you could on the wards and it gives you the opportunity to gain access to patients with rare and uncommonly seen conditions.

Which revision course should I do?

As with anything in life, there is a great deal of variability in the quality and content of these types of courses. Try to look for a well-established course that has received good feedback from course attendees. Ask your friends and colleagues which courses they attended before their exams and which they would recommend. Don't book onto a course without thoroughly researching it first to ensure that it is suitable for the exam that you are sitting.

There is also a great deal of variability in the cost of these courses. Look around as the most expensive course isn't always the best one and there are some very good value courses on the market. There is no need to break the bank and unnecessarily extend your student loan further!

Look for courses that focus on your weakest areas; for example, before my MRCP PACES examination I had great concerns about the ophthalmology station and did a stand alone course focusing on this specific area. By the time I had attended the course I had gained great confidence in examining the fundus and I had turned an area of weakness into an area of strength.

Revision courses 'do's and don'ts'

Do:

- ✓ Look for a well-established course
- ✓ Pay special attention to marking schemes given out on the course
- ✓ Look for a course that focuses on an area of weakness

Don't:

- ✗ Book onto a course without researching it first
- ✗ Break the bank and overspend

Making the Most of Your Memory

"Memory is the treasure house of the mind wherein the monuments thereof are kept and preserved" – Thomas Fuller

Tricks of the mind

There are numerous methods and tricks available that you can use to help you recall information. I have tried all of the ones I will explain in this chapter with varying degrees of success. I would recommend giving each of them a go and using the methods that work best for you.

Mnemonics

Using mnemonics is one of my favourite memory tricks and has helped me remember many difficult concepts over the years. A mnemonic is a learning technique that uses a pattern of letters, ideas or associations to assist in remembering something. The word 'mnemonic' is derived from the Ancient Greek word 'mnemonikos', which means 'relating to memory'. For whatever reason, mnemonics are very commonly used in medicine and I am certain that you will have encountered several already.

Mnemonics work by translating information into a form that is more easily retained by the brain. They make material more meaningful by adding associations and creating patterns and work best for material that is less meaningful to start with. They also help to organize information so that it can be more easily retrieved later and they typically involve visualizations that help make the facts more vivid. I can still remember mnemonics now that I learned in medical school almost 20 years ago.

A simple example of a mnemonic is the phrase '**M**emory **N**eeds **E**very **M**ethod **O**f **N**urturing **I**ts **C**apacity'. This can be used to remember the spelling of the word mnemonic, with the first letter of each word in the phrase being used.

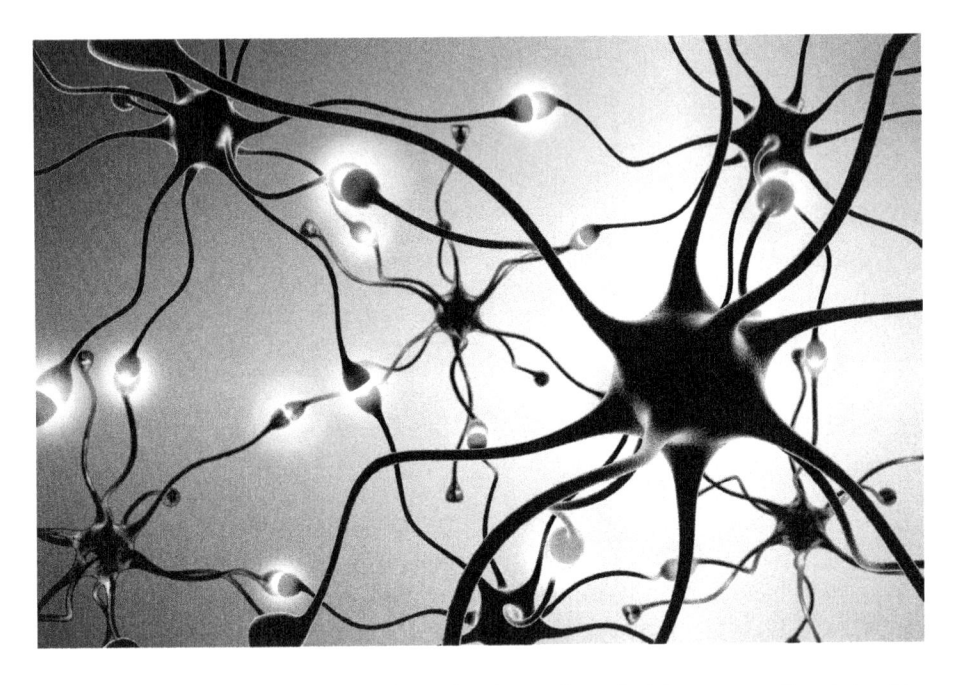

Mnemonics work by translating information into a form that is more easily retained by the brain.

One of the most commonly used mnemonics encountered in the early stages of clinical medicine is 'SOCRATES'. This mnemonic helps the student to remember the questions that they need to ask to evaluate the nature of pain that a patient is experiencing. This time each letter in 'SOCRATES' will trigger a question that should be asked to explore the patient's pain:

- **S**ite – where is the pain situated?
- **O**nset – when did the pain start?
- **C**haracter – what is the character of the pain e.g. sharp, dull etc?
- **R**adiation – does the pain radiate anywhere?
- **A**ssociations – are there any other symptoms associated with the pain?
- **T**ime course – does the pain occur at any particular times or follow any pattern?
- **E**xacerbating/ relieving factors – does anything make the pain worse or better?
- **S**everity – how severe is the pain?

There are numerous websites available with lists of medical mnemonics available, an example being http://www.medicalmnemonics.com. It can be fun to try and write your own though.

Mind-maps

Mind-maps are a visual map of your ideas, usually created around a central idea or concept. They are a fantastic way of making notes on complex information. They help you to focus on important information using key words and can be easily annotated to contain important text and diagrams. They also allow visual connections to be made and are particularly useful for visual learners.

Below is an example of a mind map that I have made around the central concept of chest pain and in particular its differential diagnosis:

Chest Pain Mind Map

CHEST PAIN

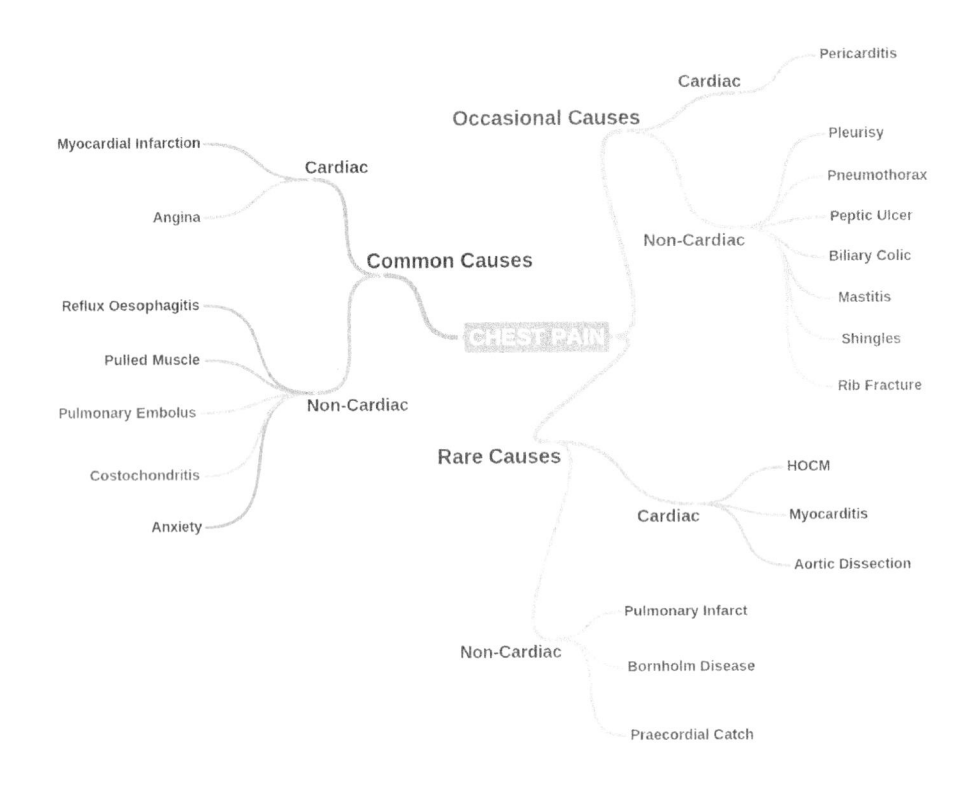

- **Common Causes**
  - Cardiac
    - Myocardial Infarction
    - Angina
  - Non-Cardiac
    - Reflux Oesophagitis
    - Pulled Muscle
    - Pulmonary Embolus
    - Costochondritis
    - Anxiety

- **Occasional Causes**
  - Cardiac
    - Pericarditis
  - Non-Cardiac
    - Pleurisy
    - Pneumothorax
    - Peptic Ulcer
    - Biliary Colic
    - Mastitis
    - Shingles
    - Rib Fracture

- **Rare Causes**
  - Cardiac
    - HOCM
    - Myocarditis
    - Aortic Dissection
  - Non-Cardiac
    - Pulmonary Infarct
    - Bornholm Disease
    - Praecordial Catch

Many studies have shown the usefulness of mind-mapping for students and one particular study (Cunningham et al 2005), showed that 80% of students thought that 'mind-mapping helped them to understand concepts and ideas in science'.

Method of loci

Method of loci, more commonly referred to as the mind palace technique, is a method used to help memorize large chunks of information. If you are a fan of the TV show 'Sherlock' you will have seen Sherlock Holmes use this technique to seek and reassemble important facts and associations in his memory to help him solve 'The Hounds of Baskerville' case.

The mind palace technique works as follows:

1. Firstly visualize a place, this could be a room or a building. Make a mental image of what you see in the room or within the building.
2. Then make a mental connection between one of these images and a manageable chunk of information. For example if you see a table you could associate this with a list of investigations needed or the differential diagnoses for a particular medical condition.
3. When you need to recall this information, perhaps in the exam itself, retrace your steps around the room until you find the table or any other item that you have used to connect information to. This should act as a trigger to remember the information connected with that particular object.

Mind palaces have been used effectively for centuries and there is documentation of it being used as a memory technique in Roman and Greek times. It is also used by memory expert Derren Brown to perform amazing feats of memory such as memorizing the order of 20 packs of cards in under an hour. Give it a try and see if it works for you.

Rhyming

Turning important pieces of information into rhymes is another great way of making the information easier to remember. It works in a similar way to building a mnemonic by creating easy to remember associations in your memory.

An example of a memory rhyme is the following traditional rhyme used to remember how many days there are in each month:

> '*Thirty days have September,*
> *April, June, and November.*

All the rest have 31,
Except for February all alone,
It has 28 each year,
but 29 in each leap year.'

Rhyming is an excellent learning method for auditory learners. Why not see if you can come up with a rhyme about a difficult to remember piece of information that relates to the exam that you are sitting?

Which memory tricks should I use?

Play around with these techniques, some will work particularly well for you and others might not. Try to focus on the techniques that you feel work best and don't get too bogged down using those that don't.

Key points to remember:

- ✓ Utilise the various memory tricks available to improve your learning
- ✓ Try creating your own mnemonics
- ✓ Mind-maps are an excellent tool for visual learners
- ✓ Large chunks of information can be learned using 'mind palaces'
- ✓ Rhyming is a useful tool for auditory learners

PART 3

UNDERSTANDING YOUR EXAM

Understanding the Syllabus

"Read the syllabus you must." – Yoda

Make sure you read the syllabus!

Earlier in this book, in the preparation and planning chapter, I stated that 'the syllabus should be the centrepiece of your exam preparation and may well be the most important single document that you read.' I believe in this so strongly that I have added an entire chapter explaining why I think that this is the case and how to make the most of using the syllabus.

What is the syllabus?

The syllabus is an outline of the content of the course or exam that you are sitting. It will have been prepared by the medical school or college that has set the exam, with the aim of providing specific guidance on the information needed to successfully pass the exam. The syllabus is thought to be so important that some university courses now set a quiz on the syllabus to encourage students to read it.

It also serves to ensure that everyone sitting the exam has an equal and fair understanding of what the exam content will be. Therefore, if you haven't read the syllabus you will be at a huge disadvantage compared with another student that has.

How to read the syllabus

I would recommend reading the syllabus from cover to cover initially to gain a good overview of the knowledge that is needed for your particular exam. Then return to the syllabus and divide the major topics into three 'traffic light' groups:

- Green - Topics that you have a good understanding of;
- Amber - Topics that you are familiar with but require more work;
- Red - Topics that are unfamiliar to you and are likely to require the most work

Once you have the syllabus areas divided into these three groups you should then incorporate them into your revision timetable, allocating the most time to the topics you are unfamiliar with and the least time to those that you have a good understanding of.

Key points to remember

- ✓ It is vitally important to read and understand the syllabus
- ✓ The syllabus is an outline of the content of the course or exam that you are sitting
- ✓ Use the syllabus to help plan your revision timetable
- ✓ Allocate the most revision time to the topics you are unfamiliar with

Understanding the Language

"The chief virtue that language can have is clearness, and nothing detracts from it so much as the use of unfamiliar words." – Hippocrates

The subtleties of medical linguistics

Medical language and terminology can be extremely challenging to understand and convey. Listening to a group of doctors talking amongst themselves can be mystifying for a layperson.

Medical language has its origins in Greek, Latin and also the modern national languages. The majority of influential medical journals are currently written in English, and English has become the language of choice at international conferences.

Having a solid understanding of medical terms that commonly occur in exams can prevent the candidate from misunderstanding a question and as a consequence answering that question incorrectly. Most medical students and doctors have a strong grasp of disease names, drug names and most commonly used medical terminology but the confusing manner in which questions are often asked still catches some out.

In this chapter I will list and explain some of the terms that commonly occur and that can cause confusion.

Commonly encountered medical exam terms

Abnormality:
An abnormality is an abnormal feature, characteristic or occurrence. In the clinical setting this generally refers to a pathologically relevant clinical feature or the result of an investigation that lies outside of the standard deviation of the population being studied.

Always:
There is a saying that there is 'no always or never in medicine'. The definition of always is 'that something occurs at all times or on all occasions'. It is very unusual for the statement that something 'always' occurs to be correct, particularly in the setting of a multiple choice style question.

Assessment:
An assessment, or clinical assessment, usually refers to the complete work-up of a patient, including history taking, physical examination and the use of investigations.

Asymptomatic:
A disease is considered to be asymptomatic when a patient has the disease but experiences no symptoms. The term clinically silent is also sometimes used. Hypertension is a classic example of an asymptomatic disease.

Borderline:
Borderline usually means that something is only just acceptable or only marginally belongs to a category. A borderline case may not be clearly classifiable.

Brand name of a drug:
The brand name of a drug is the name chosen by the manufacturer. There can be several brands of the same drug. A brand name is also

called the proprietary name. The brand name should not be confused with the drug class name or the generic drug name.

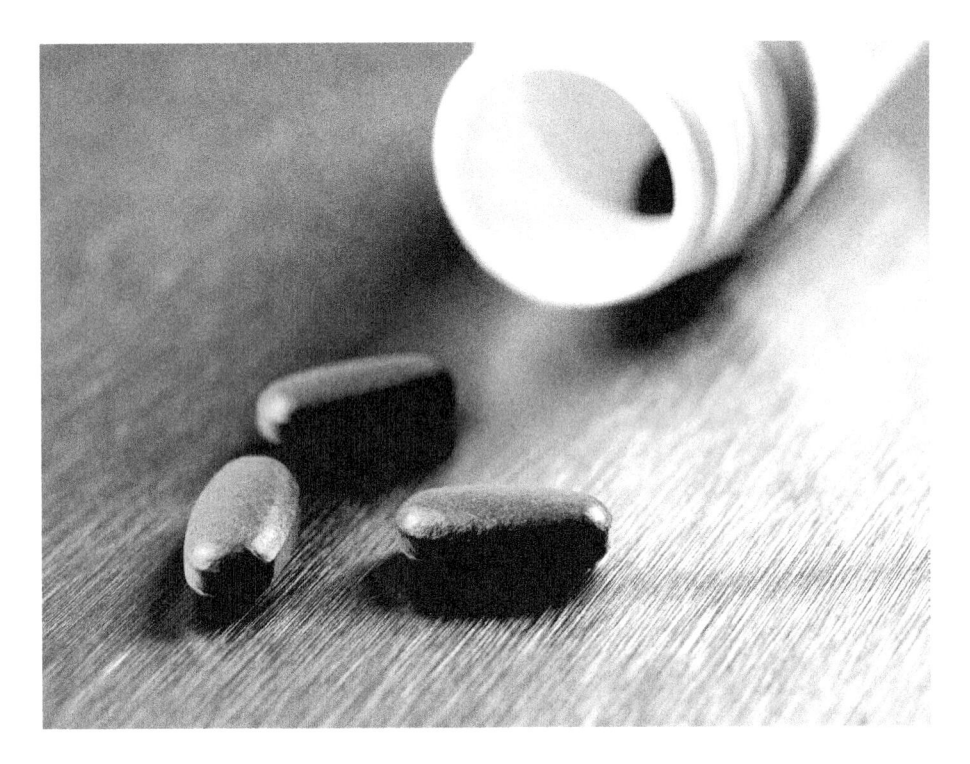

Do not confuse the brand name of a drug name with the generic name.

Characteristics:
A characteristic generally refers to a distinguishing feature or attribute of a medical condition. You should expect the characteristic to be consistently present in that condition. For example right iliac fossa tenderness is characteristic of appendicitis.

Class of drug:
A drug class is a group of drugs that have something in common. They are usually similar in some way, but they are not identical. They may be related by their chemical structure, the fact that they work in the same way or because they are used for the same purpose. This should not be confused with the generic name or brand name of a drug.

Clinical findings:
The clinical findings are any abnormalities discovered during the clinical assessment including symptoms, signs and vital signs. It does not, however, include the results of any investigations performed.

Commonly or commonest:
The use of the word commonly or commonest in a question usually indicates that something occurs in greater than 75% of the population being referred to. It may also mean that something has a greater than 75% incidence or prevalence. For example, the statement that autoimmune disease is commonest in women indicates that more than 75% of patients suffering with autoimmune disease are women.

Condition:
Condition, or medical condition, is a broad term used that includes all medical diseases and disorders.

Criterion and criteria:
A criterion is a principle or standard by which something can be judged or assessed. In the medical setting it is generally used to refer to an aspect of a formal national guideline or scoring system. Each criterion can be a clinical sign, observation or the result of an investigation that can help to assist in the formulation of a management plan for a patient. For example, the Glasgow Coma Scale (GCS) is a well-known neurological scoring system that aims to provide a reliable way of recording the conscious state of a person for initial as well as subsequent assessment. The patient is assessed against the criteria of the scale, and the resulting score gives a numerical value for their level of consciousness.

Definitive management or treatment:
This generally refers to the management or treatment that is necessary to provide a cure for a condition. It can include medical and surgical management. It may also refer to the gold standard treatment that is accepted as providing the best results for managing the condition in question.

Describe:
If asked to describe something in an exam you should give a detailed account of the subject, including a description of the appearance and characteristics of the subjects. It is often worthwhile including relevant negatives.

Differential diagnosis:
A differential diagnosis is a list of the most probable underlying causes for a set of clinical symptoms and signs. For example, the differential diagnosis of vertigo would include labyrinthitis, vestibular neuritis, benign positional vertigo, Ménière's disease and vertebrobasilar ischaemia.

Discuss:
Candidates are sometimes asked to discuss a scenario or a problem in written exams and vivas. A discussion should include an examination of the advantages and disadvantages of the particular alternatives asked for on the subject that is being discussed.

Disposition:
This refers to the location a patient is sent to following treatment in an Emergency Department, outpatient clinic or ward. Examples would include a patient being discharged home from a clinic, admitted to a hospital ward from an Emergency Department or admitted to an Intensive Care Unit from a ward.

Epidemiology:
The study of the incidence, distribution, causes and effects of health and medical conditions within defined populations.

Essential management or treatment:
This usually refers to life saving management or treatment steps that are the primary priority. It does not include investigations or non-essential treatments. An example of an essential treatment would be the administration of adrenaline (epinephrine) to a patient in anaphylactic shock.

Factor:
A factor in the setting of a medical exam usually refers to an influence or element that contributes to the development of a condition.

Feature:
A feature is a distinctive attribute or aspect discovered in the medical history, physical examination or investigations. Clinical features can be both symptoms and signs.

Generic name of a drug:
This is defined as a drug product that is comparable to a brand/reference listed drug product in dosage form, strength, quality and performance characteristics, and intended use. It has also been defined as a term referring to any drug marketed under its chemical name without advertising. The generic names for drugs are chosen by a variety of official bodies. Generic drug names can vary from country to country: for example, the generic name for one common pain medication is acetaminophen in the USA. However, in many other countries, such as the UK, the same drug is called paracetamol.

Gold standard test:
The gold standard test is the best available diagnostic test to which all other tests can be compared. An example of a gold standard test is a CT pulmonary angiogram for the diagnosis of a pulmonary embolus. Gold standard tests tend to change over time as medical science advances.

History:
The information gained by a physician by asking a set of specific questions to a patient. One common convention is to subdivided the history into the following sections:

1. Presenting complaint
2. History of the presenting complaint
3. Past medical history
4. Drug history

5. Allergies
6. Social history
7. Family history
8. Systems review

Incidence:
A statistical measure of the risk of developing a condition within a specified period of time. Incidence is equal to the number of new cases over a set time period divided by the population size.

Interpret:
If asked to interpret a set of findings or results you are generally being asked to make a diagnosis or create a differential diagnosis.

Investigations:
Investigations refer to any tests that are used to assist the process of making a diagnosis or monitoring a patient's condition. These include blood tests, ECGs, radiological investigations, biopsies, microscopy, cultures and endoscopic investigations.

List:
If asked to create a list you should create a sequence of numerically ordered or bullet pointed connected items, one below the other.

Management:
The management of a patient includes all aspects of the patient's care. This would include the patient's treatment, supportive measures used in their care and the patient's disposal. It would also include investigations that can result in an immediate change in the treatment protocol, for example checking an arterial blood gas level in a patient with COPD to assist with oxygen titration.

Most likely:
This is often used in multiple-choice questions or best answer questions when more than one of the available alternatives is

correct. For example, if you are asked for the most likely cause of a community acquired pneumonia and the choices include *Steptococcus pneumoniae*, *Mycoplasma pneumoniae* and *Legionella pneumophila*, all would be a possible cause but *Steptococcus pneumoniae* would be the 'most likely' cause.

Never:
There is 'no always or never in medicine' – see 'always'.

Outline:
If asked to outline something you should make a brief description of the subject.

Pathophysiology:
The combination of the pathology and physiology that together explains the processes and mechanisms by which a medical condition develops and progresses. If asked to describe the pathophysiological sequence of events you should attempt to list the events that occur on a cellular and physiological level in time order. For example in the development of diabetic ketoacidosis the pathophysiological sequence of events could be described as follows:

1. Absolute insulin insufficiency
2. Excess production of counter-regulatory hormones (glucagon, growth hormone, catecholamines)
3. Poor glucose utilization by peripheral tissues
4. Increased triglyceride breakdown into free fatty acids
5. Increased glucose production from hepatic gluconeogenesis
6. Beta oxidation of the free fatty acids into ketone, acetoacetate and beta-hydroxybutyrate
7. Resulting in ketoacidosis and hyperglycaemia
8. Dissociation of ketoacids into hydrogen ions and metabolic acidosis

Pathognomonic:
A clinical feature that is characteristic of a particular disease. These can be both symptoms and signs. An example would be Koplik's spots inside the mouth, which are pathognomonic of measles. Pathognomonic signs have very high specificity for a diagnosis, but do not necessarily need to have a high sensitivity. (see specificity and sensitivity)

Prevalence:
A statistical measure which demonstrates the proportion of a population that is found to have a condition within a set time period.

Precipitating cause or factor:
An agent, event, condition or characteristic that plays an essential role in the development of a disease state. For example, recognized precipitating factors for an Addisonian crisis include infections, injury, burns, surgery, pregnancy, anaesthesia and hyper-metabolic states.

Proprietary name:
The proprietary name of a drug is the name chosen by the manufacturer. Also referred to as the brand name. The proprietary name should not be confused with the drug class name or the generic drug name.

Protocol:
A system or set of instructions on how to deal with a particular situation or illness. These are created locally but based on accepted national guidance. They can vary greatly between countries and departments.

Rarely or rare:
The use of the word rarely or rare in a question usually indicates that something occurs in less than 10% of the population being referred to. It may also mean that something has a less than 10% incidence or prevalence. For example, venous thromboembolism is a rare side effect of the combined hormonal contraceptive pill.

Recommended:
The recommended management or treatment is the accepted best management or treatment advised by a national guideline or local protocol.

Symptoms:
A feature of a disease that is noticed by the patient and is indicative of the disease.

Signs:
An abnormal finding or characteristic discovered during the physical examination of a patient. This may include abnormal observations and vital signs.

Systems review:
Also referred to as the review of systems (ROS) or systems enquiry. This is the part of the history taking process whereby a structured, systematic evaluation is made of the symptoms perceived by the patient according to the organ systems.

Treatment:
The particular steps undertaken to cure or stabilize the patient's condition. This does not include investigations.

Usually or usual:
The use of the words usually or usual in a question normally indicates that something occurs in greater than 90% of the population being referred to or on greater than 90% of occasions. For example, a deep vein thrombosis is the usual cause of a pulmonary embolus.

Vital signs:
These are measures of basic bodily functions that are taken to assess the general physical health of a patient. Also referred to as the observations or 'obs'. The four primary vital signs are body temperature, blood pressure, heart rate and respiratory rate. Oxygen saturations are sometimes also included as part of the vital signs.

Key points to remember:

- ✓ Understanding medical terminology can prevent answering questions in the wrong way
- ✓ Familiarise yourself with Latin and Greek word origins
- ✓ Familiarise yourself with the terms listed in this chapter to make sure you are not caught out in the exam
- ✓ There is 'no always or never in medicine'!

Understanding Acronyms and Abbreviations

"brb, ttyl ok? Wow, I saved a 'ton' of time with those acronyms." –
Stephen Colbert

Acronyms and abbreviations in medicine

Acronyms are abbreviations formed from the initial components in a phrase or a word. These are usually presented as individual letters. Acronyms are very commonplace in medicine and many of them are entirely unique to the medical world. They add a further layer of complexity to medical language and to cause further confusion, some of them are derived from Latin.

There is often an appendix added to exam papers with a list of acronyms that may be encountered in the exam and what they stand for. In this chapter I provide a table of some of the commonest acronyms that you are likely to encounter in your medical exams. I hope that you find it a useful reference tool.

Acronym:	Meaning:
AAA	Abdominal aortic aneurysm
ABG	Arterial blood gas
ACE	Angiotensin converting enzyme
ACL	Anterior cruciate ligament
ACJ	Acromio-clavicular joint
ADH	Anti-diuretic hormone

Acronym:	Meaning:
ADHD	Attention deficit hyperactivity disorder
AF	Atrial fibrillation
AIDS	Acquired immune deficiency syndrome
ALP	Alkaline phosphatase
ALS	Amyotrophic lateral sclerosis
ALT	Alanine aminotransferase
AMD	Age related macular degeneration
AST	Aspartate aminotransferase
AVM	Arterio-venous malfomation
AXR	Abdominal X-ray
bid / bd	*'bis die'* in Latin. Means to take twice daily
bds	*'bis die sumendum'*. Twice daily (as above)
BMI	Body mass index
BP	Blood pressure
BPH	Benign prostatic hyperplasia
BRCA	Breast cancer gene
BUN	Blood urea nitrogen
CA	Cancer
CABG	Coronary artery bypass graft
CAD	Coronary artery disease
CCF	Congestive cardiac failure
CD	Controlled drug
cf	*'confer'* in latin. Means to compare to.
CF	Cystic fibrosis
CHD	Coronary heart disease or congenital heart disease
CHF	Congestive heart failure
CK / CPK	Creatine kinase / creatine phosphokinase
CNS	Central nervous system
COPD	Chronic obstructive pulmonary disease
CPR	Cardiopulmonary resuscitation
CRF	Chronic renal failure
CRP	C-reactive protein
CSF	Cerebrospinal fluid

Acronym:	Meaning:
CST	Continue same treatment
CT	Computerized tomography
CVA	Cerebrovascular accident
C-spine	Cervical spine
CXR	Chest X-ray
D&C	Dilatation and curettage
DIB	Difficulty in Breathing
DIC	Disseminated intravascular coagulation
DM	Diabetes mellitus
DVT	Deep vein thrombosis
Dx	Diagnosis
DW	Distilled water
ECG / EKG	Electrocardiogram
ECHO	Echocardiogram
EEG	Electroencephalogram
EMG	Electromyogram
ENT	Ear, nose and throat
ERCP	Endoscopic retrograde cholangiopancreatography
ESR	Erythrocyte sedimentation rate
ESRD	End-stage renal disease
et	'et' in Latin means and
FSH	Follicle stimulating hormone
GI	Gastro-intestinal
GIT	Gastro-intestinal tract
GFR	Glomerular filtration rate
GORD / GERD	Gastroesophageal reflux disease
GU	Genito-urinary
HAV	Hepatitis A virus
Hb / HGB	Haemoglobin
HBV	Hepatitis B virus
HCT	Haematocrit
HCV	Hepatitis C virus
HDL	High density lipoprotein

Acronym:	Meaning:
HIV	Human immunodeficiency virus
HRT	Hormone replacement therapy
HTN	Hypertension
hs	'*hora somni*' in Latin means at bedtime
IBD	Inflammatory bowel disease
IBS	Irritable bowel syndrome
ICD	Implantable cardioverter defibrillator
ICP	Intracranial pressure
ICU	Intensive care unit
ID	Intradermal
IDDM	Insulin-dependant diabetes mellitus
IM	Intramuscular
IN	Intranasal
INR	International normalized ratio
IP	Intraperitoneal
IT	Intrathecal
IU	International unit
IUD	Intra-uterine device
IV	Intravenous
IVP	Intravenous pyelogram
IVU	Intravenous urogram
JVP	Jugular venous pressure
LDL	Low density lipoprotein
LFT	Liver function test
LMN	Lower motor neurone
LP	Lumbar puncture
LVF	Left ventricular failure
LVH	Left ventricular hypertrophy
mane	'*mane*' in Latin means early or early in morning
mdu	'*more dicto utendus*' in Latin means at bedtime
MI	Myocardial infarction
mitte	'*mitte*' in Latin means to send
MMR	Measles, mumps and rubella (vaccination)

Acronym:	Meaning:
MRI	Magnetic resonance imaging
MRSA	Methicillin resistant *Staphylococcus aureus*
MS	Multiple sclerosis
NG	Nasogastric
NIDDM	Non insulin dependant diabetes mellitus
NKDA	No known drug allergies
nocte	*'nocte'* in Latin means at night
NS	Normal saline
NSAID	Non-steroidal anti-inflammatory drug
OA	Osteoarthritis
OCD	Obsessive compulsive disorder
od	*'omne in die'* in Latin means every day
om	*'omne mane'* in Latin means every morning
on	*'omne nocte'* in Latin means very night
OPD	Outpatient department
PAD	Peripheral arterial disease
PET	Positron emission tomography
PFT	Pulmonary function test
PID	Pelvic inflammatory disease
PMS	Premenstrual syndrome
PR	*'per rectum'* in Latin means via the rectum
po	*'per os'* in Latin means by mouth or orally
prn	*'pro re nata'* in Latin means as needed
PSA	Prostate specific antigen
PT	Prothrombin time
PTH	Parathyroid hormone
PTSD	Post traumatic stress disorder
PTT	Partial thromboplastin time
PUD	Peptic ulcer disease
PV	*'per vaginum'* in Latin means via the vagina
PVC	Premature ventricular contraction
PVD	Peripheral vascular disease
qd	*'quaque die'* in Latin means every day

Acronym:	Meaning:
qds	'*quater die sumendus*' in Latin means four times a day
qid	'*quater in die*' in Latin means four times a day
qqh	'*quater quaque hora*' in Latin means every four hours
RA	Rheumatoid arthritis
RBC	Red blood cell
Rx	Treatment or prescription - derived from the Latin '*recipe*'
SAD	Seasonal affective disorder
SIDS	Sudden infant death syndrome
sig	'*signa*' in Latin means directions
SLE	Systemic lupus erythematosus
SOB	Shortness of breath
stat	'statim' in Latin means immediately or without delay
STD	Sexually transmitted disease
STI	Sexually transmitted infection
T3	Triiodothyronine
T4	Thyroxine
TAH	Total abdominal hysterectomy
TB	Tuberculosis
tds	'ter die sumendum' in Latin means three times a day
TFT	Thyroid function test
TIA	Transient ischemic attack
TIBC	Total iron binding capacity
tid	'ter in die' in Latin means three times a day
TMJ	Temporo-mandibular joint
TSH	Thyroid stimulating hormone
TURP	Transurethral resection of the prostate gland
UMN	Upper motor neurone
ung	'*unguentum*' in Latin means ointment
URTI / URI	Upper respiratory tract infection
USS	Ultrasound scan
ut / ud	'ut dictum' in Latin means as directed
UTI	Urinary tract infection
WBC	White blood cell

Acronym:	Meaning:
WCC	White cell count
XR	X-ray
XRT	Radiotherapy

Key points to remember:

- ✓ Abbreviations are used very commonly in medicine
- ✓ Acronyms are abbreviations formed from the initial components in a phrase or a word
- ✓ Familiarize yourself with the acronyms and abbreviations in the above table to make sure you are not caught out in the exam

Understanding the Questions

"The art and science of asking questions is the source of all knowledge." – Thomas Berger

Which question types are most commonly encountered?

Whilst there are a great number of different ways of testing medical students and doctors in exams, the most commonly encountered question types are:

1. Multiple true false questions (MTFs)
2. Single best answer questions (SBAs)
3. Multiple best answer questions (MBAs)
4. Extended matching questions (EMQs)
5. Short answer questions (SAQs)
6. Essay questions

Each of these question styles has their own unique idiosyncrasies and requires a different approach and strategy.

Multiple true false questions (MTFs):

Multiple true false questions (MTFs), also often referred to as simply multiple-choice questions (MCQs), are a very commonly encountered question style. Historically they are probably the most common question type in medical exams but they have fallen out of favour over recent years and have been replaced by 'best answer' style questions in many exams. MTFs are an excellent way of testing direct factual recall and can also be used to test for recall of more obscure knowledge. They are a less reliable way of assessing higher order problem solving.

MTFs usually have a stem, which is a statement or a phrase, followed by between three and five options. An example of a typical MCQ is shown below:

Question:

Regarding aortic stenosis:

    A. The murmur is loudest in the right 2nd intercostal space
    B. An ejection click indicates supra-aortic stenosis
    C. There is a narrow pulse pressure
    D. There may be a systolic thrill best felt at the end of inspiration

Answer:

    A. True
    B. False
    C. True
    D. False

These questions can be 'positively' or 'negatively' marked and each of these requires a slightly different strategy.

When an MTF exam is positively marked it is vitally important to answer all of the questions, as you will not be penalized for incorrect answers. In a positively marked MTF guesswork alone should result in a score of 50%. The pass mark is usually set around the 70 to 75% mark, which means that you need to know the answer to half of the questions and guess 50% of the remaining questions correctly to pass.

Negatively marked MTFs must be approached with caution, as each incorrect answer will result in the loss of a mark. The pass mark in these types of MTF exams is usually much lower. In a negatively marked MTF exam try to go through and answer the questions you know the answer to first. Then re-review and attempt the others once you have done this.

If time allows, review the questions and answers again after finishing the exam as it is possible that you may have misread some questions on the first attempt. When you are unsure of the answer it is usually best to stick to your first instinct and not be tempted to change the answer on re-reading.

Single best answer questions (SBAs)

Single best answer (SBA) questions are probably the most common question style currently encountered in medical exams. They require convergent thinking and the ability to come up with a single answer to a set problem. It is easier for the examiner to test higher order thinking, such as application and evaluation of knowledge, in a SBA than in a MTF question.

Standard format SBA questions usually have three parts:

1. A statement or a clinical scenario that the question will be asked about
2. The question itself
3. The answer options, which will include one single correct answer

An example of a standard SBA question is shown below:

Question:

A 42-year-old African-American woman presents complaining of headaches, blurred vision and intermittent central chest pain for the past couple of weeks. Her fundoscopic examination reveals retinal haemorrhages and bilateral papilloedema. Her initial observations are as follows: HR 89, BP 228/134, SaO$_2$ 98% on air, BM 8.2, GCS 15/15.

Which of the following is the SINGLE most likely diagnosis?

- A. Acute myocardial infarction
- B. Pulmonary embolus
- C. Idiopathic intracranial hypertension
- D. Intracranial neoplasm
- E. Malignant hypertension

Answer: E. Malignant hypertension

The answer options will contain one single correct answer and several other distracting options. The question commonly asks for the 'single most likely diagnosis' or the 'most appropriate next management step'. In many SBA questions several of the answer options are correct, but only one will be the 'best' answer.

I generally read the question first, which allows me to see what the main emphasis of the question is. I then scan the answers, so that I know what particular kind of answer is required. Finally I read the statement or clinical scenario at the start of the question.

Within the statement or clinical scenario there will be useful clues to point you towards the correct answer. It is worthwhile highlighting or underlining these clues whilst reading the scenario. Most clinical scenarios will include vital signs, history points, examination findings and/or results of investigations. I tend to highlight any of these that are abnormal. Sometimes there are also images of investigations to interpret, such as X-ray or CT scans. Each of these will have been included for a reason so pay careful attention to what they show.

In addition to the correct answer, each SBA question will usually contain at least one or two answers that are highly unlikely or obviously wrong. There are then often one or two answers that are plausible and these serve as the main distracters within the question. Cross out and eliminate the answers that are obviously incorrect so that you have narrowed your choices.

A good way of practicing SBA questions in the run up to an exam is to cover up the list of answers and attempt to formulate an answer without the options to guide you. By attempting to remember key facts from your memory in this way you can augment your ability to recall the information later.

I wouldn't recommend using this strategy in the exam though, as on the day itself you will need every advantage that you can get!

Some SBAs require multiple cognitive steps in order to reach the correct answer. These sorts of questions are used to discriminate the best candidates. Typically you will be required to make a diagnosis and choose an answer based upon this diagnosis. An example of this sort of SBA question is shown below:

Question:

A 62 year-old woman presents with worsening shortness of breath, hoarseness of her voice and pain radiating down the medial side of her right upper arm into her forearm and hand. She is a long-term smoker and suffers with COPD. On examination she has weakness and noticeable wasting of the muscles of her forearm and hand. Her chest X-ray is shown below:

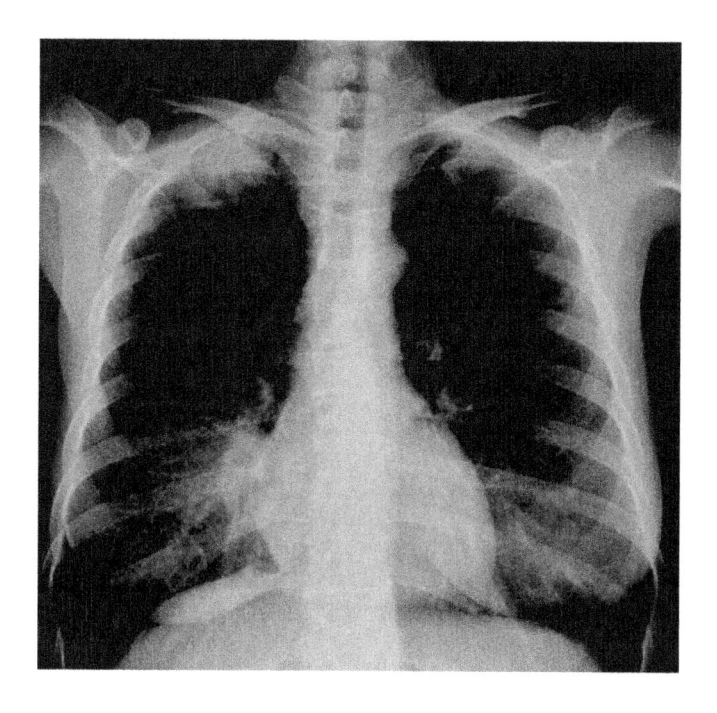

Image sourced from www.wikipedia.org

Which of the following clinical signs is MOST likely to also be present in this patient? Select ONE answer only.

- A. Left-sided pupillary miosis
- B. Right-sided pupillary mydriasis
- C. Left-sided ptosis
- D. Right-sided anhydrosis of the forehead
- E. Right-sided exophthalmus

Answer: D. Right-sided anhydrosis of the forehead

To answer this question correctly the candidate first has to recognise that there is a large mass at the apex of the lung that is most likely to be a squamous cell carcinoma. She has ipsilateral shoulder and arm pain, wasting of the intrinsic hand muscles and parasthesia on the medial side of the arm.

She also has a hoarse voice, which is likely to be caused by compression of recurrent laryngeal nerve. From this, the candidate should be able to work out that the unifying diagnosis in this case is Pancoast syndrome, which is often accompanied by Horner's syndrome caused by compression of the sympathetic chain from the hypothalamus to the orbit. The three cardinal features of Horner's syndrome are ipsilateral ptosis, pupillary miosis and anhydrosis of the forehead. Therefore, after several cognitive steps the candidate can arrive at the correct answer.

You can see by following the clues in the scenario in a stepwise and logical fashion, the correct answer can be logically arrived at even in these more challenging questions.

Multiple best answer questions (MBAs)

Multiple best answer (MBA) questions are very similar to single best answer questions, but instead of there being one answer that is correct there is more than one correct answer.

Just like SBA questions, MBA questions usually have three parts:

1. A statement or a clinical scenario that the question will be asked about
2. The question itself
3. The answer options, which will usually include two or three correct answers

An example of a standard MBA question is shown below:

Question:

You are a doctor working on an elderly care ward. One of your patients is an 82-year-old woman with a lower respiratory tract infection. Her condition has deteriorated overnight and it seems unlikely that she will survive much longer without intensive care input. She has been assessed by a member of the intensive care outreach team, who has stated that she is not a suitable candidate for an ICU admission because of her significant co-morbidities and poor likelihood of survival. Her husband is the listed next of kin. He is, however, quite frail and suffers with Parkinson's disease, which causes him to have some mobility difficulties. You also have the contact details of a family friend. A nurse on the ward has asked you to contact her family and/or friends.

Which of the following would be the most appropriate course of action? Select the TWO MOST appropriate options.

- A. Argue with the ICU team and insist that she is admitted
- B. Contact the family friend and ask them to pass on the information to the husband
- C. Contact the husband by telephone and inform him of the severity of his wife's condition
- D. Call for an ambulance to collect the husband immediately
- E. Suggest that the husband attends hospital soon with some family or friends for support
- F. Wait for a few more hours before doing anything to see if there is any change in her condition
- G. Call for a taxi to collect the husband

Answer:

- **C. Contact the husband by telephone and inform him of the severity of his wife's condition**
- **E. Suggest that the husband attends hospital soon with some family or friends for support**

When approaching MBA type questions it is important to prioritize the most likely or most important answers. Sometimes a mark is awarded for each correct choice but sometimes all of the answers need to be correct in order to score a mark.

In this particular question some of the answer choices are clearly incorrect. It is obviously an inappropriate use of the emergency services to collect the husband and bring him to hospital, it is also not your responsibility to call a taxi or arrange transport for him at this point in time. Arguing with the ICU outreach team, who have considerable expertise in the management of these types of patient, would also be highly inappropriate. Waiting to see what will happen will waste valuable time and run the risk of the husband not being able to spend time with his wife before her death. By asking the family friend to contact the husband you would be breaching confidentiality so this is also not appropriate.

Contacting the husband and informing him of the severity of his wife's condition is clearly very important at this stage and he should be able to make a decision himself on whether to visit. If further help with regards to transportation is needed this could be addressed during this phone call. Suggesting that he has some support would be very sensible, especially in view of his Parkinson's disease and frailty.

Once again, by approaching the question a stepwise and logical fashion and using a process of elimination the two most appropriate answers can be easily arrived at. It could even be argued that someone without a medical background could correctly answer this question, simply by using a common sense approach.

Extended matching questions (EMQs)

Extended matching questions (EMQs) first appeared in 1993 after work by Case and Swanson. They have become an increasingly popular way of testing medical students and doctors over the past few years. MCQs and SBAs have received some criticism as it has been suggested that candidates can often guess the answer via a combination of what they partially know and utilization of clues in the question. It has been suggested that EMQs address some of these key flaws and are a better means of assessing higher knowledge as opposed to simple factual recall.

A standard EMQ generally has four parts:

1. A theme that sets the stage for the questions
2. A list of options from which the questions that follow can be answered
3. A lead-in that gives the candidate instructions on how to answer the questions
4. The questions, usually in the form of clinical scenarios but can also be statements of facts or data that requires interpretation

An example of an EMQ is shown below:

Theme: Tropical diseases

Options:

- A. Malaria
- B. Typhoid fever
- C. Meningitis
- D. Shigellosis
- E. Ebola virus disease
- F. Cholera
- G. Giardiasis
- H. Anthrax
- I. Salmonella food poisoning
- J. HIV infection
- K. Dengue fever
- L. Polio

For each of the clinical scenarios below select a **SINGLE MOST** likely diagnosis from the list above. Each option may be used once, more than once or not at all.

Question 1: A 38-year-old attended a wedding 24 hours ago. At the wedding they ate a chicken dish, and there have been at least 20 people that have been unwell subsequently. She presents with a fever and crampy lower abdominal pain. She has had six episodes of bloody diarrhoea.

Question 2: A 56-year-old gentleman recently returned from a trip to Liberia where he was helping with a health relief agency. He returned 2 days ago and is now complaining of feeling very weak and has severe diarrhoea and vomiting. He is also complaining of a sore throat and noticed that his gums bled this morning when brushing his teeth.

Question 3: A 25-year-old woman has recently returned from her travels in Canada, where she was on a canoeing trip on the Ontario Lakes. She presents with diarrhoea that she has had for over a week. She has no temperature, but does feel a little nauseous and she has lost around 3kg in weight.

Question 4: A 19-year-old woman has returned from her GAP year in Mozambique where she has spent 6 months helping in a rural school. She is complaining of feeling intermittently very hot and then shivering intensely, and her bed is often drenched with sweat at night.

Question 5: A 21-year-old woman returned from a holiday in Indonesia one week ago. About 14 days ago she had met up with a group of friends and they had eaten a lot of shellfish. 4 days ago she started to develop diarrhoea, but now is complaining of constipation. She also feels hot and sweaty and has noticed a rash on her arms. Whilst she is in your surgery, you note that she has a dry cough.

Answer 1: I. Salmonella food poisoning
Answer 2: E. Ebola virus disease

Answer 3: G. Giardiasis
Answer 4: A. Malaria
Answer 5: B. Typhoid fever

It can be seen that this EMQ is testing the candidates knowledge of a wide spectrum of infectious diseases and requires a greater knowledge base to answer all five parts than an MCQ or SBA would require. Distracters have been included to attempt to increase the complexity of the question and to help discriminate the better candidates. The difficulty in this particular question has been further increased by the fact that the same answer can be used more than once, increasing the number of potential answers for each part and removing the ability of the candidate to exclude options by a process of elimination.

It is a good idea to read all five questions and attempt to formulate an answer for each without the options as guidance. If you then can see your proposed answer in the list of options you can answer with a greater degree of confidence. EMQs generally require a good understanding of the topics the question is assessing and are probably the most discriminatory method of testing the candidate in a multiple choice or multiple option type question style.

Short answer questions (SAQs)

Short answer questions (SAQs) require the ability to formulate an answer based on the information given in the question without the advantage of having options to choose from. They usually take the form of a clinical scenario and often contain data that requires interpretation such as a list of blood results, X-rays, ECGs or rhythm strips. There will then be a list of questions that require knowledge about the subject matter presented in the clinical scenario.

They are less commonly encountered than the multiple choice, probably because they cannot be marked by an automated machine and require a real examiner to assess the results. The answers to the questions are usually agreed upon by a board of examiners before the examination. Additional answers encountered in the marking process can be added to the marking scheme if they hadn't been thought of initially and they are agreed to be appropriate by the examining board. For this reason they are an excellent means of assessing candidates but require a great deal of input.

An example of an SAQ is shown below:

Question:

A 65 year-old man presents with a week's history of palpitations. His past medical history includes a previous stroke 2 years ago, hypertension and type 2 diabetes. His current medications are ramipril, metformin and aspirin. He has no known drug allergies and is a non-smoker. His initial observations are: HR Approximately 130 bpm (irregular), BP 145/90, temperature 36.9°C. His rhythm strip is shown below:

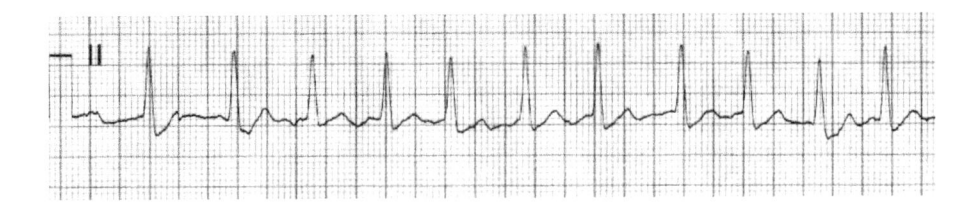

(a) What is the diagnosis? (1)
Atrial fibrillation

(b) List 4 potential causes of this condition. (2)
- Hypertension
- Pulmonary embolism
- Coronary artery disease
- Other primary heart disease e.g. HOCM, congenital etc
- Hyperthyroidism

- Alcohol
- Drug abuse e.g. cocaine
- Sepsis / infection

(c) Name an oral medication that could be used as first line treatment for rate-control in this gentleman. (1)
Beta-blocker e.g. bisoprolol or;
Calcium channel blocker e.g. diltiazem

(d) List 3 factors that would make a rate-control strategy preferable in his long-term management. (3)
Any three of:
- Age over 65
- Presence of coronary artery disease
- Contraindications to anti-arrhythmic drugs
- Unsuitable to cardioversion e.g. contraindications to anticoagulation or structural heart disease
- Long duration of AF (> 12 months)
- Absence of congestive heart failure

The best way to answer SAQs is with short answers that are to the point and with bullet-pointed lists for the questions that require more information to be presented. By using sentences and paragraphs of information it makes the answers more difficult for the marker to see. Bullet points present the information in a very clear manner and increase your chances of picking up the marks available.

The first part of a SAQ is often the diagnosis, and although often only worth 1 mark, this is clearly a very important part of the question and getting it wrong can mean that all subsequent parts of the question will be incorrect as a consequence. In this question there is a short clinical scenario followed by a rhythm strip that demonstrates that the patient is in atrial fibrillation. The rest of the question asks about the causes and first-line treatment of this condition. The last part of the question is usually the most challenging part and requires either higher knowledge or understanding of a national guideline or protocol.

SAQs are an easy way to test data interpretation and also the understanding of scoring systems and key guidelines. It is therefore advisable to look through the syllabus and see what sorts of investigations, guidelines and scoring systems are most likely to come up, and ensure that you have a detailed understanding of them.

Essay questions

Essay questions are probably the most challenging question type for both the candidate and the examiner. For this reason it is unusual to encounter them in medical examinations. They do still come up from time to time though and I will run through a strategy with which to approach them here.

Time management is essential with essay questions, so try to allocate time for each of the following steps according to the length of the exam. Take the first 5 to 10 minutes or so of the exam to plan ahead, read the question thoroughly, preferably twice during this time, to ensure that you are answering the right question in the right way. Even a slight misreading or misinterpretation of an essay question can be completely disastrous. You are being asked a specific question that will require a specific answer that is related to it.

The next step should be allocated to 'brainstorming'. Jot down all of the ideas and information that pops into your head with regards to the question being asked. I tend to use a mind-map approach to this, as outlined in the 'Making the Most of Your Memory' chapter earlier in this book. I place the essay title or question at the centre of my notes page and then radiate the ideas outwards around it. This is the easiest way for you to get your thoughts onto paper in an organized manner in the shortest possible time.

Now that you have brainstormed, you need to organize your ideas into a well-structured essay. Try to split the essay into ordered sections and write a paragraph or two in each of these sections. Most essays need to be sandwiched between an introduction and a conclusion or discussion that summarizes the main points.

Try to make the essay easy to read, and if lists of information are required makes these bullet pointed. If the style of essay required allows for it, have clearly underlined headings that catch the examiner's eye that make it transparent what you are writing about in each section.

Finish with a good conclusion that summarizes the main points and arguments that you have laid out in the essay.

If you know that your exam will contain an essay question you should dedicate a good proportion of your study time to writing essays under timed conditions. Practicing in this manner will make the process much less stressful on the examination day and will improve your time management considerably.

Key points to remember:

- ✓ There are 6 common question types that appear in medical exams
- ✓ MTFs tend to test direct factual recall
- ✓ SBAs, MBAs and EMQs are better at testing higher-order knowledge
- ✓ Be succinct and use bullet points when answering SAQs
- ✓ Practice essay writing under timed conditions

Understanding OSCEs

"Practice does not make perfect. Only perfect practice makes perfect." – Vince Lombardi

What are OSCEs?

OSCEs, or objective structured clinical examinations, are designed to test the theoretical knowledge and clinical skills of medical students and trainee doctors. They test a wide variety of skills including history taking, physical examination, communication skills and the ability to perform practical procedures.

OSCEs were originally described by Harden et al in 1975 and have grown in popularity tremendously over the past decade or so, almost completely replacing the more traditional clinical examinations where a candidate is escorted around a series of patients by an examiner. Studies have shown that OSCEs are an effective tool for evaluating the areas that are most critical to the performance of doctors.

An OSCE usually consists of a circuit of stations, each of which is between 10 and 20 minutes long. Each station will test a different skill or competence and is usually invigilated and marked by a different examiner or examiners. Candidates rotate around all of the stations sequentially so that each candidate will have had a standardized experience.

OSCEs are designed to be:

1. Objective: Each candidate will be exposed to identical stations marked by the same examiner or examiners. There is generally a

fixed marking scheme, which the examiners adhere to. The goal is that the examination is as free from bias as is possible and therefore the exam is fair, impartial and gives each candidate equal opportunity for success.

2. Structured: The stations are arranged to cover a wide variety of skills, with each station examining a different skill. Most OSCEs are very carefully organised in order to cover a specific skill set that is required by the medical student or doctor sitting them. A great deal of planning and preparation goes into the setting of OSCEs so that they are as close a representation of real life clinical practice as possible.

3. Clinical examinations: OSCEs attempt to re-create the feel of actual clinical practice. In a typical OSCE the candidate will encounter a sequence of scenarios and skill stations that mimic the conditions of a working clinician. I have heard OSCEs described by some as a 'bad day at the office'. They examine the candidate's ability to perform the skills required by a doctor under stressful circumstances.

The importance of practice

Preparing for an OSCE is a very different process from preparing for a theory based multiple choice or written examination. There are a wide variety of resources available explaining the ideal way to take histories, undertake systems examinations and perform the specific technical skills that are commonly encountered in OSCEs. Some books and revision courses also contain model marking schemes and these are especially helpful. Marks will be awarded for each step in the particular task that you have been asked to perform, and knowing what the marks are awarded for makes it far easier to pass the station. It is essential to learn the correct methodology for each of these and practice each of them repetitively until they are second nature to you. The importance of this type of repetitive practice cannot be emphasized enough.

Practice in small groups with your friends and colleagues, and take it in turns to role-play the candidate, patient and examiner. It is very helpful to get used to being the examiner as you can gain a useful insight into the sorts of mistakes that can easily be avoided and see where easy marks can be picked up by monitoring and marking the performance of your colleagues. When practicing in this manner, try to simulate the feel of the examination as closely as possible. Pay careful attention to time keeping as it is very common for candidates to run out of time, particularly in history taking and communication skills type stations. If possible, also try to get experienced senior clinicians, preferably with some experience of marking or invigilating OSCEs, to watch you. Many useful tips can be picked up in this way.

Some OSCEs will have life support or resuscitation type stations that will require the demonstration of advance life support, advanced pediatric life support or advance trauma life support skills. Try to get hold of the hospital resuscitation officer or a senior Emergency Room doctor to help you with practicing these types of scenarios. Some hospitals have dedicated simulation labs where these skills can be practiced in circumstances that closely resemble real life and these provide an excellent environment in which to practice and hone these types of skills.

When practicing with your friends and colleagues, ask them to not be overly friendly and even ask them if they can harass you a little and ask difficult or awkward questions. Also be very critical and analytical of each other's performance. By practicing all of the skills that you require for your OSCE in this manner you will develop a familiarity with the kind of stress that these examinations generate and this familiarity will help you enormously on the day of the exam when your nerves are at their peak.

Presentation skills

Presentation of your findings is a key part of most OSCE stations and marks are often weighted to represent this. At the end of many OSCE stations a short concise presentation will be required summarizing the important findings and outlining a diagnosis and brief management plan. It is vitally important to spend time preparing your presentation skills. The more you practice presenting in this manner, the slicker and more professional you will appear and the more likely you are to pick up the marks available for this part of the station.

Before you start your presentation take time to carefully consider what you say. Maintain good eye contact with the examiner during the presentation and speak in a clear articulate manner without mumbling. Stand tall, hold your stethoscope gently in front of you, and avoid fidgeting with your hands or stethoscope. Never guess or make up a diagnosis and if you are not sure let the examiner know this. Honesty is always the best policy and guessing is a sure fire way to create problems. If you have said something that you subsequently realize is incorrect, apologize to the examiner and explain that it was said in error. Under no circumstances argue with an examiner.

When listing a differential diagnosis, try to start by listing the commonest and most likely diagnosis first. Have a clear and logical thought process for listing the differential, for example use the well known surgical sieve method.

When presenting in front of the patient, always be tactful and considerate of their feelings. Avoid using terms such as 'cancer', which could be potentially very upsetting to the patient, and instead use terms such as 'neoplastic disease'.

When you know the diagnosis and are confident in your findings, demonstrate this to the examiner by speaking in a forthright and confident manner. Your confidence will send the message that you are a competent clinician that is safe to pass this exam and move on to the next stage of your medical training.

General tips for how to approach the OSCE

Your own personal presentation is very important, so dress neatly and professionally. Cut your nails and comb or brush your hair and tie any long hair back. There are no marks provided for your appearance but it will send a message to the examiner that you are taking the exam process seriously.

Some OSCEs will have a set dress code so make sure you have read the exam guidance before you arrive. Under most circumstances a short-sleeved shirt or blouse, open at the neck, or a long-sleeved shirt or blouse with the sleeves rolled up in combination with smart trousers or a skirt will be most appropriate. The usual convention in current clinical practice is for the arms to be bare below the elbow, with no watches or jewellery to be worn on the hands or wrists (with the exception of a wedding band), for the purposes of infection control and hygiene. Most hospitals have also outlawed the wearing of ties for the same reason. This dress code should be adopted in OSCEs also and shows a good understanding of modern clinical practice.

Knock on the door before entering the room and greet the patient in a professional manner, introducing yourself by name and clarifying your position. For example, 'My name is Joe Smith and I am a medical student undertaking my final examinations.' Make physical contact with the patient by shaking hands and ask them for their name. Explain to them what you have been asked to do and why you are doing it. Say please and thank you and remain polite at all times. Maintain good eye contact with the patient and do not attempt to communicate with them out of the role that they have been asked to play. When communicating with patients, speak clearly and avoid medical jargon. If the patient has any questions or concerns, acknowledge these and attempt to answer the questions or address their concerns as best as possible. Be direct and honest but also remain sensitive.

Your interaction with the examiner should be limited to explaining what you are doing, if that has been asked for, presenting findings in your summary and answering any questions that they have asked you. If the examiner has asked you a question that you don't know the answer to, do not be tempted to guess or make something up as this will raise questions about your probity and your ability to know your own limitations.

If there are written instructions about the station, read them very carefully and mentally prepare yourself for the task that lies ahead. If these instructions are given verbally, then listen carefully and ask for the instructions to be repeated if you are not 100% sure what you have to do. There are no marks given for history taking in examination stations and vice versa, so only do what the instructions ask for.

If possible, wash your hands at the beginning and end of every station. There are usually marks available for doing this and these marks can make the difference between a pass and fail when your performance has been borderline. Remain in the room for the allotted time period and close the encounter when signalled to do so. At the end of the station thank the patient, as they are often real patients that have given up their time to be there. It is a good idea to thank the examiner too as this will be the last impression they get of you before awarding the final marks for the station. Leave the station when instructed to do so by the examiner and not before.

Try to remember that in most OSCEs the examiners are looking for competence, not excellence, from the candidate. They want to see a doctor that has a patient centered approach, who can be trusted to look after patients in a real world clinical setting.

Broadly speaking, there are 5 types of station that are commonly encountered in OSCEs:

1. History taking stations
2. Clinical examination stations
3. Communication skills stations
4. Practical skills stations
5. Data interpretation stations
6. Teaching stations

1. History taking stations

History taking stations in OSCEs serve to assess the candidate's ability to explore the patient's presenting complaint and gather pertinent information based on this presenting complaint. They also assess the candidate's ability to communicate with the patient, formulate a management plan based upon the history and enter into a discussion about the history with the examiners.

When taking a history from a patient, particularly in an exam scenario, it is important to make the patient feel as comfortable as possible. You should sit at the same level as the patient and not stand above them. Try to sit with an open posture with your arms uncrossed and avoid leaning forwards into the patient. Candidates often feel uncomfortable taking a history whilst being watched by an examiner, so it is a good idea to focus your full attention on the patient and act as you would do in an unobserved clinical setting. Practicing taking histories with people watching will help you to become more adjusted to this.

Use open-ended questions and avoid questions that can be answered with a simple 'yes' or 'no'. Avoid asking multiple questions at the same time in 'machine gun' fashion as this will confuse the patient and make it difficult for you to extract the most important points from the history. The use of short pauses in between questioning can be helpful to ensure that the patient has fully expressed everything that they wish to say.

Many of the patients that you encounter in history taking stations will not be actual patients but instead professional actors and actresses that have been trained and prompted to give a medical history in a certain fashion. These actors and actresses tend to be very consistent in their answers between candidates and are often very skilled in the use of body language, emotional and personality characteristics. Look carefully for any non-verbal cues that might be being offered by them. The patient or actor in these stations sometimes has the ability to award points for how they feel the candidate has performed, so it is important remain polite and to attempt to develop a rapport with them during the station.

Here is an example of a typical history taking station that may be encountered:

HISTORY TAKING STATION – Patient that is seeing flashing lights

Information for the candidate:

Bob Jones is a 55-year-old man that has presented seeing flashing lights. Please take a history from the patient as appropriate.

Information for the patient (actor):

The candidate is a final year medical school student taking their final exams. They have been asked to take a history from you and will be assessed upon their ability to do so. Do not simply read out the information that has been given to you but instead wait for the candidate to ask you specific questions and then answer the questions as appropriate.

Your name is Bob Jones and you are a 55-year-old man that works as an IT consultant. You have been seeing flashing lights on the outer aspect of your vision for the past 24 hours.

You have no eye pain, photophobia, eye redness or discharge from the eye. You feel that your vision is reduced in your right eye and that there is a 'dark shadow' moving across your field of vision in that eye. You are also seeing 'floaters', which have a 'cobweb' like appearance.

You are not experiencing any other significant symptoms, such as facial pain or headache and there is no history of a foreign body in the eye or any eye trauma.

You are short-sighted and usually wear glasses but have no history of any previous eye problems.

You have a history of diabetes mellitus, which developed 6 years earlier. You take metformin 500 mg three times a day for this. You take no other medications and have no known drug allergies. You have never had any surgery or previous hospital admissions. Your mother suffered an eye problem, but you are unsure exactly what it was and do not know how it was treated.

You are a non-smoker but drink alcohol a few times per week. You currently consume approximately 20 to 25 units of alcohol per week.

At the end of the history taking process please ask the candidate what they think is wrong and what is going to happen next?

Information for the examiner:

In this station you should assess whether the candidate is competent to take a full and accurate history from the patient, generate a differential diagnosis and answer a few brief questions about their differential diagnosis.

At the start of the station you should instruct the candidate to 'take a history from this patient, establish a differential diagnosis and outline a brief management plan to include any further examination or investigations.'

An appropriate differential diagnosis would be:

- Retinal detachment
- Posterior vitreous detachment
- Vitreous haemorrhage

Further investigations and management should include:

- Check patients visual acuity
- Dilate pupil and perform a fundoscopic examination
- Ocular ultrasound scan could confirm diagnosis of retinal detachment
- Patient should be referred urgently for a specialist ophthalmology opinion

Marking sheet:

	Achieved	Not achieved
Appropriate introduction to patient		
Confirms patients name and age		
Confirms patients occupation		
Elicits presenting complaint		
Discusses history of presenting complaint		
Asks about eye pain		
Asks about discharge		
Asks about time of onset		
Asks about floaters		
Asks about visual loss		
Asks about any history of trauma		
Asks if patient has had headache		
Asks if patient has had facial pain		
Asks if any previous eye problems		
Asks if patients wears glasses or contacts		
Asks about PMH (diabetes mellitus)		
Asks about drug history (metformin)		
Checks if patient has any drug allergies		
Asks if any family history of eye problem		
Discusses social history		
Performs a systems review		
Generates appropriate differential diagnosis		
Asks if can check visual acuity		
Explains further eye examination needed		
Answers patient's questions appropriately		
Presents a clear summary		
Discusses clear management plan		
TOTAL SCORE:		/ 27

2. Clinical examination stations

Clinical examination stations assess the candidate's ability to perform a thorough, stepwise examination routine. They usually also assess the candidate's ability to interpret the clinical signs elicited during the examination.

At the start of the station you should engage with the patient and fully explain what you are planning to do in the examination. Expose all of the areas required for the particular examination routine that you have been asked to perform, but always ask for the patient's consent before doing this and use the patient's gown to cover the patient and maintain their dignity. Properly position the patient on the examination table before starting; for example, sit the patient up at a 45° angle for a cardiovascular examination. If you have forgotten to perform part of the examination, simply go back and do it at the end. It does not usually matter which order things are performed in as long as they are done at some point.

If you have been asked to perform an examination of a sensitive or personal area, such as a breast examination, explain to the patient why it needs it be done and offer for a chaperone to be present. Be courteous and helpful to the patient throughout the examination and help them on and off the table and assist them with dressing and undressing if it is required. Be gentle with the patient at all times and never hurt them, look at the patient's face during palpation and ask them to let you know if they are experiencing any discomfort during the examination. Hurting a patient will almost certainly lose you marks and may even result in you failing the station.

Here is an example of a typical physical examination station that may be encountered:

CLINICAL EXAMINATION STATION – Cardiovascular examination

Information for the candidate:

Ethel Jones is a 70-year-old woman that has been experiencing increasing shortness of breath over the past few weeks. Please perform an examination of her cardiovascular system and then present your findings to the examiner.

Information for the patient:

During this station the candidate will perform an examination of your heart and chest. You will be positioned lying flat on the couch, but the candidate may ask you to sit up or re-position you.

You should not answer any questions from the candidate about your history or diagnosis. If the candidate requires any further information during this station the examiner will provide it.

Information for the examiner:

In this station you should assess whether the candidate is competent to perform a thorough and logical cardiovascular examination, generate a differential diagnosis and answer a few brief questions about their differential diagnosis.

At the start of the station you should instruct the candidate to 'perform a cardiovascular examination on the patient, establish a differential diagnosis and outline a brief management plan to include any further examination or investigations.'

The patient in this particular station has an ejection systolic murmur that radiates to the carotids and is consistent with a diagnosis of aortic stenosis. Please examine the patient before the exam starts to ensure that you are familiar with the clinical signs present in this patient.

An appropriate differential diagnosis would be:

- Aortic stenosis
- Aortic sclerosis

Further investigations and management should include:

- ECG (looking for signs of LVH)
- Chest X-ray (looking for post-stenotic aortic dilatation)
- Echocardiography (to confirm the diagnosis)
- Patient should be referred for a specialist cardiological opinion

Marking sheet:

	Achieved	Not achieved
Washes hands / hygiene measures		
Appropriate introduction to patient		
Obtains consent to perform examination		
Sits patient up to 45-degree angle		
Appropriately exposes chest		
Inspects from the end of the bed		
Examines both hands		
Feels radial pulse for rate and character		
Asks to check blood pressure		
Feels brachial and carotid pulse		
Inspects neck and assesses JVP		
Inspects chest, looking for scars etc		
Palpates apex beat		
Checks for heaves and thrills		
Auscultates all 4 cardiac areas		
Auscultates apex in left lateral position		
Auscultates aortic area sitting forwards		
Auscultates axilla for MR radiation		
Auscultates neck for AS radiation (present)		
Auscultates lung bases for crepitations		
Palpates liver for pulsation		
Feels lower limb pulses		
Checks for peripheral oedema		
Presents a clear summary		
Correct diagnosis of aortic stenosis		
Discusses clear management plan		
TOTAL SCORE:		/ 26

3. Communication skills stations

Communication skills stations assess the candidate's ability to communicate with both patients and colleagues in a variety of challenging and often emotionally taxing circumstances. An increasing emphasis on good communication skills has been seen in medical training over the past two decades and it is now a major part of most medical school and postgraduate medical exam syllabi.

Unlike the history taking and clinical examination stations, there is no set routine that can be followed and the process is much more fluid and unpredictable. Because of this unpredictability, candidates often dread these stations.

Commonly encountered communication skills scenarios include:

- Breaking bad news
- Explaining a procedure
- Obtaining consent
- Family planning
- Genetic test counselling
- Confidentiality issues
- Safeguarding children and vulnerable adults
- Advanced directives
- Dealing with complaints
- Dealing with difficult patients and relatives
- Dealing with difficult colleagues

Each of these scenarios comes with its own set of unique problems and issues that need to be dealt with, but there are a few basic principles that you can follow to improve your performance. Make sure that you have carefully read the prompt and understand what you have to discuss properly before you start. Ensure that the area is private and that you are using appropriate body language. Just as in the history taking station, you should sit at the same level as the patient with an open posture. Attempt to make a connection with the patient, maintain good eye contact and give the patient your undivided attention. Remain polite and empathetic at all times. If you are dealing with an angry patient remember that this may be a coping mechanism that is helping them to deal with a difficult situation and it is not a personal attack on yourself. Likewise, if you are dealing with a difficult or aggressive colleague do not be drawn into an argument, and remain calm and collected. The examiners will be looking for a doctor that acts in a professional manner.

Probably the commonest scenario that arises in communication skills stations is the breaking of bad news. This can occur in a variety of ways, varying from the communication of a diagnosis of cancer, passing on an HIV positive test result or communicating to a relative that a loved one is terminally ill or has passed away. The SPIKES strategy outlined by Baile, W. et al. is a useful adjunct when approaching these types of station. The SPIKE mnemonic stands for:

- **S**etting
- **P**erception
- **I**nvitation
- **K**nowledge
- **E**motions
- **S**trategy & **S**ummary

The six steps of SPIKES are as follows:

Setting

Ensure that the area that you use is private and appropriate for purpose. You should be able to discuss the news with the patient without interruptions. It is often a good idea to have someone else with you, such as a nurse, when you break the bad news. Make sure that the patient has the opportunity to have a friend or loved one with them also.

Perception
Try to determine what the patient knows about their condition or the situation being discussed. Try using a 'warning shot' to see if they are prepared to receive the news.

Invitation
Once you have ascertained the patient's perception you should use a straightforward statement such as 'I have some bad news for you'. Then ask the patient directly if they want to hear this bad news. Accept the patient's right not to know if they do not want to receive the news at this point in time.

Knowledge
Avoid medical jargon and use language that is easily understood by the patient. Be direct and to the point but deliver the news in a sensitive and empathetic manner. Check whether the patient has understood what you have said and ask if they have any questions.

Emotions
Be prepared for the patient to be upset, tearful or angry and acknowledge their emotional response sympathetically. Give the patient time to express their feelings to you and try to be as supportive as possible. Offer reassurance but remain realistic and avoid giving false hope.

Strategy & Summary
Work together with the patient to develop a strategy for approaching the situation. Discuss management options and explore what the patient wants to do next. Check if they need anything clarified or any further questions answered before bringing the conversation to a close. Finally, set an agenda for the next time that you meet.

Here is an example of a typical communication skills station that involves breaking bad news:

COMMUNICATION SKILLS STATION – Breaking bad news

Information for the candidate:

You are looking after Mr. Smith, a 76-year-old man who was brought in to the Emergency Room by ambulance an hour earlier. A little earlier today he was complaining of abdominal pain and then a short while later he collapsed. He remains unconscious at this stage but is maintaining his own airway. A bedside ultrasound scan was performed, the results of which are shown below:

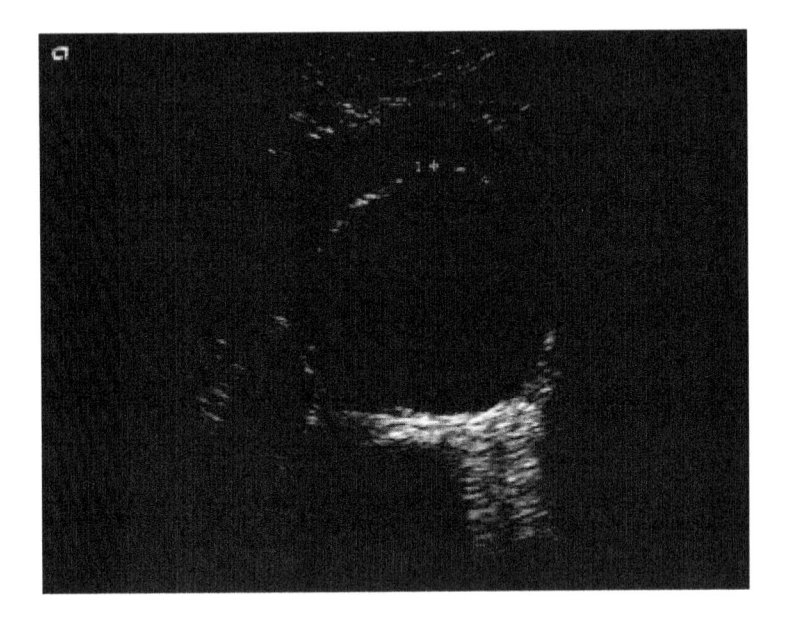

You have made a diagnosis of a ruptured abdominal aortic aneurysm (AAA) and asked for an opinion from the vascular surgeons. They have reviewed the patient and explained that he is not suitable for surgery due to his various co-morbidities. They feel that he has no chance of survival at this stage.

Mr. Smith's wife has arrived in the department and you have been asked to have a discussion with her to explain her husband's condition. Please also discuss his resuscitation status with her.

Information for the actress (Mrs. Smith):

Your husband is a 76-year-old retired builder and devout Catholic. He has a past medical history of diabetes mellitus and ischemic heart disease. He had a large heart attack earlier this year and he currently takes numerous medications. Despite this, he is reasonably active and is able to walk to the shops every day to buy his cigarettes and newspaper.

You know nothing of your husband's condition at this point in time and you are very worried about his wellbeing, having witnessed his collapse earlier.

The candidate should make his diagnosis and prognosis clear to you. You do not understand the diagnosis and ask to see the result of the ultrasound scan. The candidate may show you the scan and use this as a tool to help explain the diagnosis.

The candidate should state that he is not going to survive and also reassure you that he is not in any pain and will not experience any suffering.

The candidate should attempt to discuss your husband's resuscitation status with you and make it clear that he is not suitable for resuscitation. You do not understand why this is the case and you are concerned that he is not being treated because 'he is old'.

If the candidate does not offer, ask if you can see your husband and ask if a Catholic priest can be called for.

Information for the examiner:

In this station you should assess whether the candidate can effectively break bad news in an empathetic manner.

At the start of the station you should instruct the candidate to 'explain to Mrs. Smith about her husband's condition. Do not take a history from her about her husband.'

The candidate may choose to use the ultrasound scan picture given to explain the diagnosis to Mrs. Smith.

Marking sheet:

	Achieved	Not achieved
Candidate asks for a nurse to be present		
Appropriate introduction to patient		
Confirms name and relationship to patient		
Candidate explains his or her role		
Candidate assesses what is already known		
Uses a 'warning shot' to prepare relative		
Explains diagnosis of AAA		
Explains patient not suitable for surgery		
Explains prognosis explicitly		
Confirms understanding of prognosis		
Discusses resuscitation status		
Does not involve relative in decision		
Explains patient will not suffer		
Offers to contact friends or family		
Offers chance to see patient		
Offers to contact Catholic priest		
Uses clear language and avoids jargon		
Picks up and responds to non-verbal cues		
Allows time to react (uses silence)		
Acknowledges emotions and uses empathy		
Uses appropriate body language		
Offers to answer questions		
Closes interview appropriately		
TOTAL SCORE:		/ 23

4. Practical skills stations

There are a wide variety of practical skills that can be assessed in OSCE stations and each skill will require repetitive practice to master the routine that is needed. The sorts of practical skills that will be expected of you will become progressively more difficult as you become a more senior clinician.

Most hospitals and universities have clinical skills laboratories available where technical skills such as phlebotomy, catheterization, suturing and the insertion of chest drains can be practiced. Spend as much time as possible practicing skills in this environment, paying particular attention to the skills that you are less familiar with performing. Make sure you have a marking scheme available when practicing these skills so that you are not missing out any important steps and introducing bad habits.

Commonly encountered practical skills stations include:

- Hand washing and 'scrubbing up'
- Blood pressure measurement
- BM measurement
- Venepuncture
- Intravenous cannulation
- Intraosseous needle insertion
- Arterial blood gas sampling
- Insertion of a central line
- Administration of an injection
- Wound suturing
- ECG recording
- Checking ankle-brachial pressure index (ABPI)
- Explaining how to use an inhaler or peak flow meter
- Urethral catheterization
- Fundoscopy
- Taking a cervical smear
- Insertion of a chest drain

- Pleural aspiration
- Basic airway management
- Endotracheal intubation
- Bag-valve mask ventilation
- Application of a plaster of Paris

Obviously, each of these procedures requires different skills and equipment and you should refer to your exam syllabus to ensure that you are familiar with the sort of procedures that you will be expected to perform.

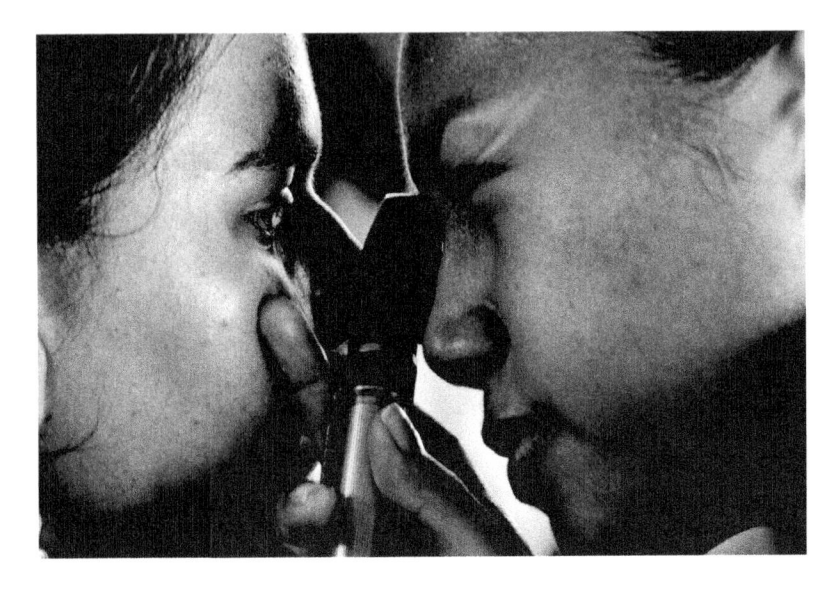

Repetitive practice should form an essential part of your preparation for practical skills stations.

When approaching any practical skills station carefully read your prompt to ensure you know exactly what is expected of you. Often there will be a patient to interact with and explain the procedure to and a separate piece of equipment to perform the actual procedure on. Although this creates a somewhat artificial situation, try to remain 'in character' and react and respond just as you would in a real-life setting. For example, if you are asked to take blood from a patient, explain to the actor that they will 'feel a sharp scratch' before you insert the needle into the venepuncture manikin arm. If there is any equipment left out for you in the station such as gloves or an apron then make sure that you use it as there will almost certainly be marks awarded for this.

Here is an example of a practical skills station that involves intravenous cannulation:

PRACTICAL SKILLS STATION – Intravenous cannulation

Information for the candidate:

In this station you must demonstrate how you would insert an intravenous cannula into a patient. An actor will be present and you should discuss the procedure with them but do NOT insert an actual needle into the actor. You will be provided with a manikin arm into which the intravenous cannula can be inserted.

Information for the actor:

During this station the candidate will insert an intravenous cannula into the mannequin arm that has been provided. They will talk to you and explain the procedure.

They have been clearly instructed NOT to insert a needle into your arm.

Information for the examiner:

In this station you should assess whether the candidate is competent to perform insertion of an intravenous cannula.

At the start of the station you should instruct the candidate to 'insert an intravenous cannula into the manikin arm that has been provided and explain the procedure to the actor provided.'

Marking sheet:

	Achieved	Not achieved
Appropriate introduction to patient		
Explains procedure to patient		
Explains may cause brief discomfort		
Gains patient's consent for procedure		
Checks has all required equipment		
Washes hands or applies alcohol sanitizer		
Applies tourniquet		
Correctly identifies vein in antecubital fossa		
Puts on gloves		
Cleans skin with alcohol wipe		
Removes cannula from packaging		
Warns patient to expect a 'sharp scratch'		
Inserts needle at appropriate angle		
Gains flashback of blood in cannula hub		
Fixes needle and advances cannula		
Releases tourniquet		
Removes needle		
Disposes needle into sharps bin		
Applies cannula dressing		
Completes and applies date sticker		
Flushes cannula with normal saline		
Disposes of gloves and equipment		
Does not ignore patient throughout		
TOTAL SCORE:		/ 23

5. Data interpretation stations

Data interpretation stations are an excellent way of assessing the candidate's clinical knowledge and presentation skills at the same time. They also assess the candidate's ability to think laterally whilst being put 'on the spot'; a very important skill for clinicians to possess.

The typical format of a data interpretation station is to be given a piece of data, often in the format of an ECG or X-ray, and then present your findings and answer questions on it.

Commonly encountered data interpretation stations include:

- Observation charts
- Fluid balance charts
- Chest X-rays
- Abdominal X-rays
- ECGs
- Blood results
- Arterial blood gas results

As with all OSCE stations, it is important to have a systematic approach and make sure that you have practiced presenting all of the commonly encountered data in your exam.

With any piece of medical data you should check that it belongs to the correct patient and was taken on the correct date. For radiological images check the adequacy of the film, paying careful attention to penetration and rotation. If presented with a set of blood results, look to see if there are reference ranges available that will give you clues about the underlying pathology. Try not to jump straight for the most obvious abnormality straight away and stick to your system so you don't overlook less obvious pathology.

Here is an example of a practical skills station that involves interpretation of a chest X-ray:

DATA INTERPRETATION STATION – Interpreting chest X-ray

Information for the candidate:

In this station you must present the provided chest X-ray to the examiner in a systematic manner, commenting on any significant changes that are present.

At the end of your presentation the examiner will ask you two questions about the X-ray.

Information for the examiner:

In this station you should assess whether the candidate is competent to interpret a chest X-ray and spot the obvious pathology that is present.

At the start of the station you should instruct the candidate to 'present the chest X-ray that has been provided' commenting on any obvious pathology.'

At the end of the station you should ask the candidate the following two questions:

1. Do you think that this X-ray should have been taken?
2. How would you manage this patient?

Chest X-ray provided for interpretation:

Patient name: Joseph Smith
DOB: 1/1/1975
Date: 1/1/2015
Erect AP film

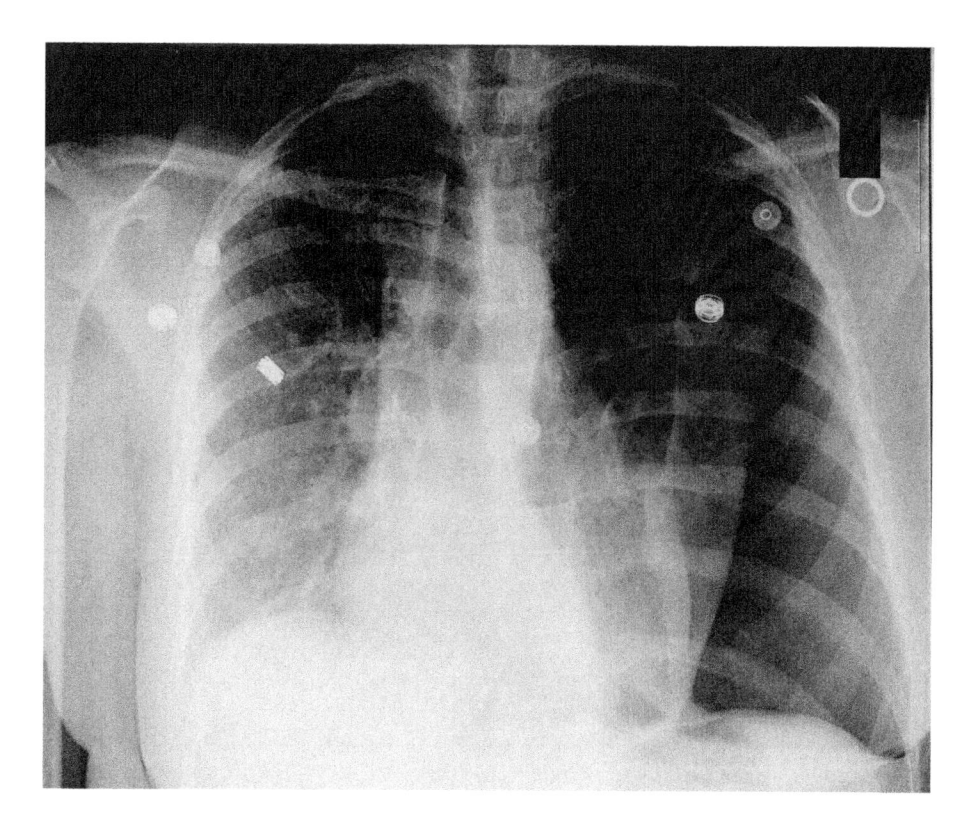

Image sourced from www.wikidoc.org

Marking sheet:

	Achieved	Not achieved
Checks X-ray belongs to correct patient		
Checks X-ray taken on correct date		
Comments on erect AP projection		
Comments on rotation		
Comments on penetration		
Comments on bony structures		
Comments on soft tissues		
Comments on position of trachea		
Comments on hilar structures		
Comments on lung zones		
Comments on costophrenic angles		
Comments on heart size and contours		
Recognizes tension pneumothorax		
Uses systematic approach to presentation		
Summarizes appropriately		
States that film should not have been taken		
Explains correct management		
TOTAL SCORE:		**/ 17**

6. Teaching stations

Teaching stations are not usually encountered until the postgraduate examination stage. Teaching is an important and often overlooked part of being a doctor and nearly all doctors are expected to teach at some point in their career. This has become increasingly recognised over recent years and teaching is now a required skill in many postgraduate exams.

Whenever you are asked to teach something in an OSCE setting, it is a good idea to start by ascertaining exactly what the student knows and what previous experience they have. You should then be able to set the objectives for the station and proceed accordingly. The student should be encouraged to ask questions throughout and you should check that they have understood what has been taught at regular intervals throughout the station. At the end of any teaching station try to summarize what has been taught.

A useful tool is the 'four-stage approach' outlined by Peyton et al. This method provides a very useful approach for teaching practical skills in simulated settings:

Stage 1
Demonstrate the skill at normal speed, silently and without any explanation.

Stage 2
Repeat the demonstration of the skill with a full explanation of each step. The student should be encouraged to ask questions during this stage.

Stage 3
Perform the skill for a third time; this time the student should provide an explanation of each step. At this point you can question the student on key issues and prompt them if they experience difficulty. You can correct the student if necessary during this stage.

Stage 4

The student performs the skills under close supervision, describing each step as they go along.

Although the 'four-stage approach' is a very useful tool for teaching, it also has its limitations, particularly in the exam setting when there is limited time available. It works best for short practical procedures, such as venepuncture or the insertion of a Guedel airway. The 'four-stage approach' is impractical when attempting to teach more complex processes, such as the interpretation of arterial blood gas results or ECGs, and when teaching these sorts of skills a question and answer approach is best, working through the process in a logical and stepwise fashion.

It is important to remember that it is your teaching style and ability that is being assessed during these stations and not your own ability to perform the procedure. With that being said, it is often very difficult to teach a procedure or skill without a good working knowledge of it.

Here is an example of a teaching station that involves teaching a medical student how to interpret an ECG:

TEACHING STATION – ECG teaching

Information for the candidate:

Please teach this third-year medical student how to perform a basic interpretation of a 12-lead ECG. Use the ECG provided and answer any questions that they put to you.

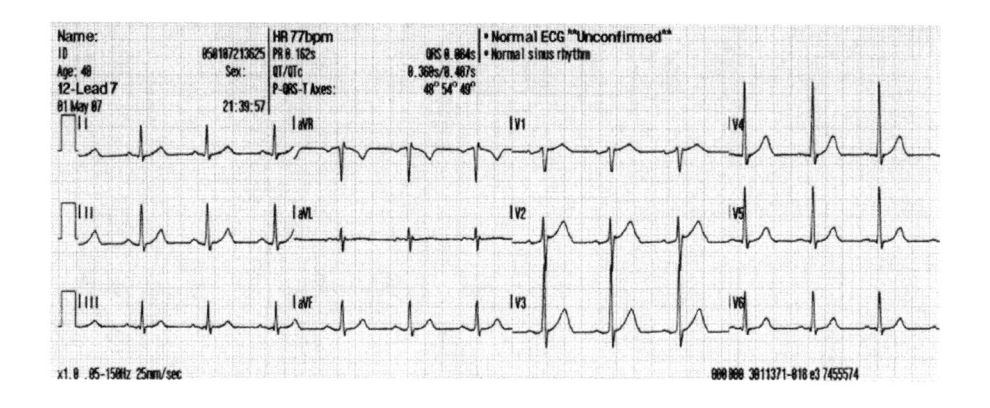

Information for the actor:

You are a third-year medical student that has some basic familiarity with ECGs but you are not confident in interpreting them. Please ask the candidate if they will explain to you how to interpret a normal ECG.

If you do not understand something ask the candidate for clarification.

You should ask the candidate two questions during the station:

1. How can I spot a myocardial infarction?
2. What is meant by a left bundle branch block (LBBB)?

Information for the examiner:

In this station you should assess whether the candidate is competent to teach a medical student how to interpret an ECG.

At the start of the station you should instruct the candidate to 'teach the medical student how to interpret an ECG using the one that has been provided.'

A piece of plain paper and a pencil have been provided that can be used to draw diagrams to assist in the teaching process.

The candidate will be asked two questions by the actor during the station and marks should be awarded only if appropriate answers are provided.

Marking sheet:

	Achieved	Not achieved
Appropriate introduction to student		
Assesses student's prior knowledge		
Explains what an ECG is in basic terms		
Basic explanation of heart electrophysiology		
Explains limb leads and chest leads		
Explains how to calculate heart rate		
Explains how to determine rhythm		
Explains how to calculate axis		
Explains P waves		
Explains PR interval		
Explains QRS complex		
Explains ST segment		
Explains T waves		
Relates above segments to cardiac cycle		
Maintains professional approach		
Checks understanding at intervals		
Uses the ECG provided to aid teaching		
Encourages questions from student		
Uses a systematic and logical methodology		
Uses diagrams to aid teaching process		
Answers first question appropriately		
Answers second question appropriately		
Summarizes for student at end		
TOTAL SCORE:		/ 23

Understanding OSCEs 'do's and don'ts'

Do:

- ✓ Dress neatly and professionally
- ✓ Practice your routines repetitively
- ✓ Use your hospital clinical skills lab to practice skills
- ✓ Remain polite and respectful throughout

Don't:

- ✗ Wear anything below the elbow
- ✗ Hurt the patient under any circumstances
- ✗ Speak before you think when presenting

Understanding Vivas

"The spoken word was the first technology by which man was able to let go of his environment in order to grasp it in a new way."
Marshall McLuhan

The dreaded viva voce

The viva voce, or oral exam, has declined in popularity over recent years but is still a part of many medical exams. It is generally the final hurdle of any particular exam and usually takes an interview style format whereby the candidate sits opposite the examiners and answers questions posed in spoken format.

It is quite different from written exams, as there is less time to think and answers cannot be returned to or re-written. There is an even greater degree of unpredictability with these exams than there is with OSCEs as there are no routines that can be practiced and very little familiar territory for the average candidate to fall back on. As well as assessing clinical knowledge, they also assess the candidate's ability to think on the spot and react under pressure; both vital skills for clinicians to possess. Even seasoned exam veterans have frozen up and gone blank in vivas. For this reason the 'viva' is probably the most dreaded of all the different types of examination that medics are faced with.

Preparing for the viva

Just like any other medical exam, preparation should start early. Try to get a feel for the sorts of questions that come up by talking to colleagues and consulting any books that might be available. Get as many people as possible to ask you viva questions under exam conditions so that you can get used to the stress and anxiety that the viva can induce.

Being videoed can be a useful way of picking up any bad habits that you have and improving your general style of speaking. I did this before one set of exams and noticed that I had a tendency to excessively move my hands around and fidget, and it assisted me in stopping this before the viva exam.

It is very common to be asked to give definitions or give lists and these should be a source of easy marks for you. These are often used as opening questions and should be second nature to you by the time you sit the viva. When reciting lists you should try to start with the commonest causes first. Think about writing flashcards with definitions and lists on that you can practice.

How to approach the viva on the day

Just as in OSCEs, personal presentation is very important. You should dress the same way that you would for a job interview, in smart but comfortable clothing. Avoid wearing outlandish ties and bright colours, such as orange and red, instead sticking to safe 'corporate colours' like navy and black. Men should wear a conventional dark coloured suit, conservative shirt and a dark coloured tie. Women should wear a conventional skirt or trouser suit and avoid low cut tops, very short skirts and excessive amounts of jewellery.

When you enter the room make good eye contact with the examiner that greets you, shake his or her hand and then ask if you may sit down. Body language is very important and sitting right back into the chair and leaning slightly forwards sends a message that you are engaged and attentive. Smile and keep your body straight and your head in a neutral position to project confidence and energy. Avoid crossing your arms and legs as this projects defensiveness. If there is more than one examiner try to engage both of them, even if only one is asking the questions.

Listen carefully to each question that you are asked and then spend a moment to think about your answer before you speak. A short pause is fine and may prevent you from blurting out the first thing that comes into your head impulsively. For example, if you are answering a question about foot injuries and start talking about metacarpals instead of metatarsals, you will cost yourself important marks. By simply taking a moment to consider what you are about to say these sorts of mistakes can easily be avoided.

Speak loudly and clearly but remain to the point and avoid waffling, the examiners are looking for a concise and logical answer, and will quickly become frustrated by unclear answers that are difficult to hear. Above all, never bluff or guess an answer; the examiners are experts in their fields and will quickly spot this.

Be prepared to answer further questions about any answer that you give. If you are asked to list the commonest causes of finger clubbing, lead with a cause that you have a good understanding of. For example it would be foolish to answer 'pachydermoperiostosis' if you know nothing about it and you would be better off answering with subject you are more likely to able to discuss, such as lung cancer or tuberculosis.

Never argue with the examiner, even if you are convinced you are correct, as many students have fallen down this way. The best-case scenario is that you are correct but you have embarrassed the examiner in the process of proving it. The worst-case scenario is that you are incorrect and have made yourself look very foolish. Instead, remain polite and courteous, and try to find another angle to approach the issue being discussed that may enable the examiner to see your point of view. Remember that the examiners are human too and that the viva is also a difficult experience for them.

If you have answered a question badly try not to dwell on it as this will distract you and may affect your ability to answer subsequent questions. Answering one question incorrectly is not a disaster but allowing it to disrupt your concentration and ability to answer subsequent questions may well be. It is also worth remembering that you may have misjudged how you answered the question and you may well have done better than you think.

At the end of viva thank your examiners and leave the room promptly. The exam is over and no more marks can be gained.

Understanding OSCEs 'do's and don'ts'

Do:

- ✓ Dress neatly and professionally
- ✓ Speak loudly and clearly
- ✓ Get as many people as possible to ask you viva questions
- ✓ Think about your answer before you speak

Don't:

- ✗ Dress in garish colours
- ✗ Use defensive body language
- ✗ Bring up topics you know nothing about
- ✗ Dwell on answers you think were incorrect
- ✗ Argue with the examiners

PART 4

THE LITTLE THINGS THAT MAKE A DIFFERENCE

Dealing With Stress and Anxiety

"Adopting the right attitude can convert a negative stress into a positive one." Hans Selye

Mental battles

Famed Endocrinologist Hans Selye, who conducted much work on stress and the human response to it, defined stress as "any event which may make demands upon the organism, and set in motion a non-specific bodily response which leads to a variety of temporary or permanent physiological or structural changes". Put in simple terms, stress is your body's way of responding to unpleasant demands.

Every student that sits an exam experiences stress and anxiety at some point. It is important to realize this and remember that you are not alone when you experience these feelings. The sheer quantity of knowledge that you are expected to learn as a medic can feel completely overwhelming at times and this in itself can be extremely stressful. Spending months locked up in a room and revising in every spare moment can cause the stress to become chronic and allow feelings of anxiety to set in.

On many occasions when preparing for exams I have personally experienced these feelings. I have allowed negative thoughts to spiral into fears of poor performance and failure. With time and experience, though, I learned to manage my stress extremely well and re-direct these feelings in a positive way that actually helped me to prepare more efficiently.

Understanding that these stresses are a normal response to your circumstances and having a basic knowledge of why you are experiencing these feelings can help you overcome them also.

Why are medical exams so stressful?

There is a tremendous amount riding on every single medical exam. When I sat the 2nd MB examination at the end of my second year in medical school it was with the knowledge that not everyone would make it through to the third year and that this would be the end of the road for some people. It had a notoriously high failure rate and, sadly, not everyone made the grade. Medical finals are the culmination of many years of hard work and study. When these have been passed, you can finally enter the medical profession as a doctor, a distinguished and respected position within society that you have been working towards your entire adult life. Passing a postgraduate exam can mean that you can enter a new job or specialty and this can have important career and financial implications. If you add all of this to the expectations that you put on yourself, and the inadvertent pressure of the expectations of family and friends, you have a perfect recipe for creating stress.

The quantity of knowledge required can also cause stress. Medicine is a vast topic and the amount that you have to learn can seem almost impossible at times. When the perceived demands upon you greatly exceed your perceived resources the stress is much more likely to feel uncontrollable.

Medical exams are also designed to be stressful, they are often considered to be a 'rite of passage' that actually assess your performance under stress. The examiners can go out of their way to make it difficult and challenging to see what you are made of. Medicine is a very stressful career and they want to see that you are the kind of individual that will be able to deal with these stresses.

Stress can be contagious too, and you should choose your study group partners cautiously. Being around an individual that is extremely stressed and having a lot of negative thoughts can easily rub off on you. I can recall one particular occasion when I was feeling fairly calm and confident about an upcoming exam. I then spent a few hours sitting and eating lunch with a friend that was extremely anxious about the same exam, and by the end of the lunch I was almost as anxious as him. Be very careful not to feed off the feelings of others around you.

After the exam can also be a very stressful time. It is tempting to sit down with others that have sat the exam and dissect the paper. It will always seem like others have answered questions in a different way or have performed better than you. There is no point in ruminating over your answers now, and what is done is done. You have finished the exam and should take some time to relax. You may have more exams in this sitting and when this is the case you should move onto the next one, putting this one behind you.

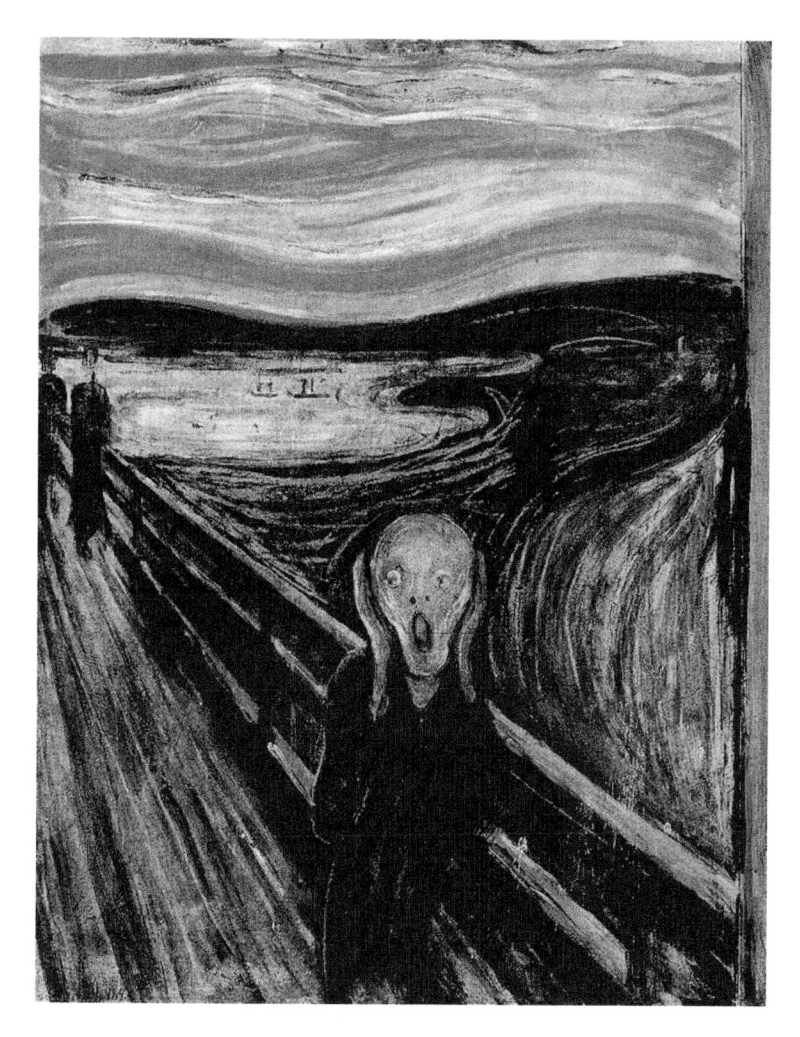

'The Scream' by Edvard Munch. Many medics feel like this in the run up to their exams!

What causes anxiety?

Anxiety is the psychological component of the 'fight or flight' response and should be considered a natural response to stressful events. It is a complex and poorly understood condition but it is widely accepted to be caused by the discharge of a variety of neurotransmitters within the sympathetic nervous system.

It is thought that there is an over-activation of catecholamines from the adrenal medulla, particularly epinephrine and norephinephrine, and an under-activation of the serotoninergic neurotransmitter system. A combination of these results in a variety of emotional symptoms including poor concentration, feelings of fear and apprehension, and physical symptoms such as dry mouth, sweating, palpitations and bowel disturbances. Anxiety can also cause poor libido, sleep disturbance and associated feelings of depression.

It is therefore not difficult to see that allowing feelings of anxiety to set in and take over can be extremely counterproductive to exam preparation!

Make exam stress your friend

Some stress is actually necessary for optimum performance. The arousal stress-performance curve first created by Yerkes and Dodson in 1908, and later adjusted by Nixon in 1979, nicely demonstrates how stress affects performance:

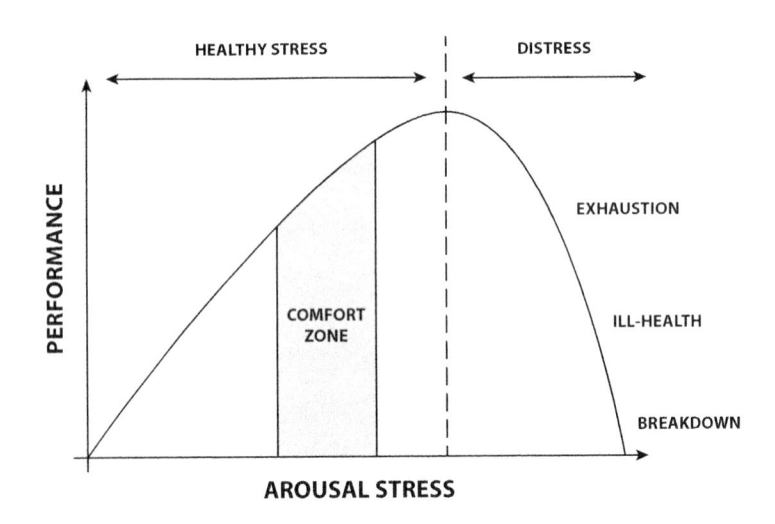

It can be clearly seen from the graph that as stress increases so does performance. This is referred to as 'healthy stress' and this is the area that you should be aiming to remain within during your exam preparation. Just above the comfort zone is a sweet spot where performance will be optimized but 'distress' has not yet been reached. After the peak of the graph performance falls off dramatically and exhaustion, ill health and eventually breakdown occur.

Try to monitor your stress levels to ensure that you are remaining in the 'healthy stress' zone as much as possible. The good news is that the curve can be shifted to the right if the correct stress management tactics are employed.

Don't make a bad situation worse

The first step to take in managing stress is to avoid things that could inadvertently make it worse. Avoid big lifestyle changes in the run up to the exam such as going on a diet or moving house. If you are planning on giving up smoking, a few weeks before the exam is not the best time to do it. If you enjoy exercising or playing sports, try to make time to continue with this, as it is likely that this is already a major stress coping mechanism for you.

Try not to disrupt the balance between the four major life areas too much. Under normal circumstances it is recommended that there is a fairly even balance between family, friends, work (this includes study) and leisure time:

WORK / STUDY	FAMILY
LEISURE	FRIENDS

Around exams it is very easy for this balance to become adversely disrupted and your study become the sole focus of your life, leaving no time for anything else:

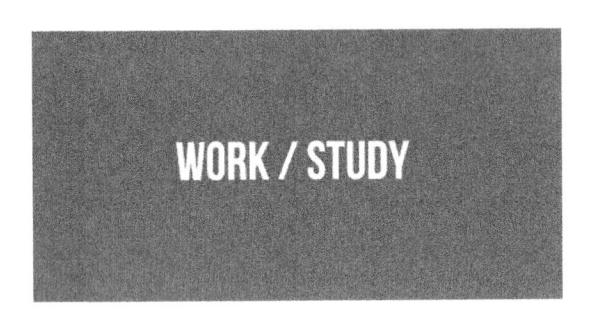

WORK / STUDY

Allotting time to all four facets of your life will keep your stress to a minimum but removing this important balance from your life will make things much worse. It is essential that your study time does not come at the expense of your family, friends and leisure time.

Stress management techniques

If you are feeling stressed and overwhelmed there are several tried and tested ways of improving the situation.

One of the most important facets of stress management is identifying the source of the stress. Much of your stress will be related to your exam preparation, but each of us has outside lives to balance as well. There may well be multiple factors contributing to the stress that you are experiencing at present and your study may well be 'the straw that broke the camels back'.

Writing a 'stress journal' can help you to identify the things that are causing you the most stress. Each time you feel stressed note it down in your journal and look for patterns that arise. Jot down what triggered the stress, how it made you feel and anything that improved it. Hopefully by doing this you can learn to avoid the situations that worsen your stress levels and raise your ability to cope with the stress that studying has caused.

If you feel extremely stressed during a particular study session, perhaps because of the complexity of a subject or simply because you feel like you are running out of time, then it is time to take a break. Trying to carry on studying whilst in this mindset is likely to be counterproductive. A change of scenery at this point in time can be very helpful and can assist with putting things into perspective. Get up and make a cup of tea, go for a walk outside or perhaps try doing some gentle exercise.

Tiredness and fatigue can increase stress and another way to reduce your stress levels is to take a short nap. A short 30-minute 'power nap' will help to recharge your batteries. There is a good reason why people in the Mediterranean take daily siestas in the afternoon. You will almost certainly feel more able to cope with an intense study session after one of these naps.

Stretching and massage therapy is another fantastic way to reduce your stress levels. Massage has additional values as well. Sitting hunched over a computer or textbook for many hours a day will increase tension in your neck and upper back and having a massage can help to significantly reduce this.

Breathing exercises can also help to reduce stress and can help you to feel calmer and more able to cope with the situation at hand. Try sitting in a warm, quite place in a comfortable chair. Relax your body as much as possible and then start to regulate and slow down your breathing. Breathe in through your nose and out through your mouth to create a 'circular pattern' to your breathing. With each in-breath visualize that you are inflating your lungs completely and with each out-breath visualize that you are emptying all of the air out. Try doing this for around 5 minutes a couple of times a day when you are feeling particularly stressed about your upcoming exam.

Dealing with stress and anxiety 'do's and don'ts'

Do:

- ✓ Stay in the 'healthy zone' on the stress-response curve
- ✓ Allot time to all the four major life areas
- ✓ Keep a stress journal
- ✓ Try breathing exercises as a form of relaxation

Don't:

- ✗ Allow yourself to enter the 'distress' zone of the stress-response curve
- ✗ Make major life changes before an exam
- ✗ 'Catch' stress from anxious study partners
- ✗ Dissect papers after you have sat them

Improving Your Confidence

"With confidence, you have won before you have started." Marcus Garvey

The importance of self-confidence

Psychologists have long reported that intelligence isn't the only predictor of academic achievement and that self-confidence is also an excellent predictor of exam success.

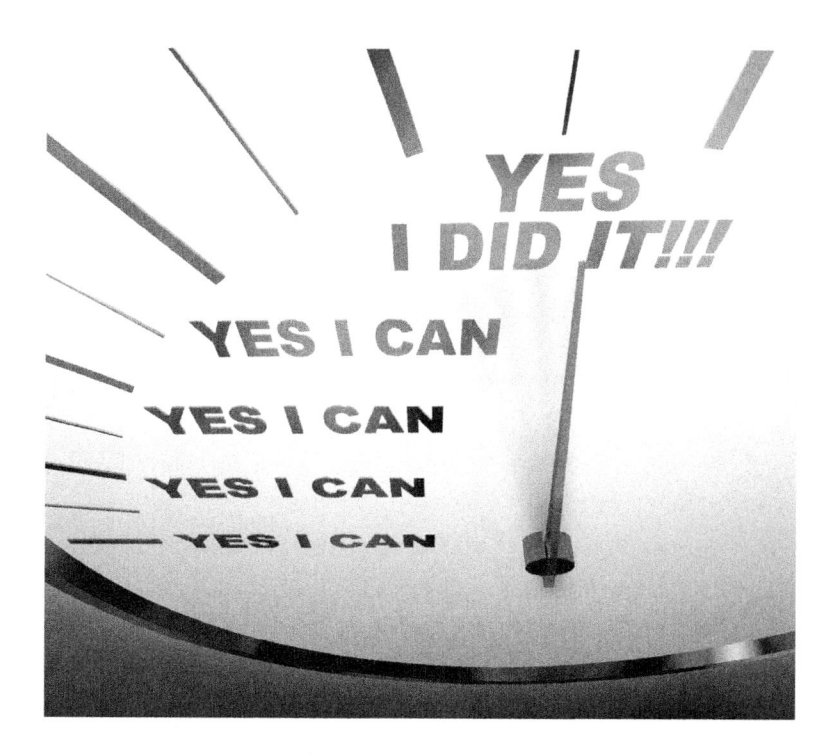

Self confidence is an excellent predictor of exam success.

One particular study by Psychologist Tomas Chamorro-Premuzic, looking at 7- to 10-year-old children, showed that the children who achieved the best marks in school tended to rate their own abilities highly and have the highest self-confidence levels.

The majority of IQs for medical students and doctors are reported to fall in the range of 105 to 135. We therefore know that intelligence is not an issue for you, and that passing these exams is well within your academic capabilities. My own experience from sitting exams has been that I have performed best when my confidence has been at its highest and this seems to have been the case with my peers also.

The power of positive thinking

Concentrating on positive thoughts and minimizing negative thoughts is a very useful method for improving your exam confidence. If you dwell on pessimistic thoughts, such as 'I am going to fail this exam' or 'my career is over if I fail this exam!', these thoughts will erode your confidence and negatively affect your performance.

Try to identify and be conscious of these thoughts and think logically about them. Are you really going to fail this exam after the 6 months of solid revision that you have done? Will your career really be over? The truth is that these scenarios almost always seem worse than they really are. The chances are that if you have prepared properly you have every chance of passing and that even if you fail you will get a chance to re-sit.

Once you have identified and challenged your negative thoughts in this way, replace them with positive thoughts. For example 'I am going to fail this exam' could be replaced by 'I am well prepared and I am NOT going to fail this exam'.

Repeat these positive thoughts to yourself during your exam preparation and even during the exam itself and you will feel your confidence grow.

Seeing is believing

Positive visualization and mental rehearsal is another way to improve your confidence and develop a positive attitude towards exams. This process has been used by athletes and sports competitors since the 1970s and is just as valid for the exam process. Consider the extraordinary boxer Muhammad Ali, considered by many as the greatest boxer of all time. He often used positive visualization techniques to enhance his confidence, and a great example of this is his epigram 'I am the greatest!'

Try using the following method for improving your confidence:

Find a quiet place, close your eyes and run through the day of the exam in your head, visualizing each step that you will go through. Watch yourself arriving for the exam and registering with the steward. You have arrived in plenty of time, you have prepared well and feel quietly confident about your chances of passing. You are ushered to your seat and sit down in the allocated place. In the countdown to the exam you organize your desk space and listen carefully to the instructions of the steward.

The bell rings and the exam starts. You open the paper and carefully read through the guidance and then the questions. You know what is required of you and have plenty of time to get through the exam. There are many familiar questions and you feel confident in your ability to answer them after your revision. Visualize yourself answering all of the questions in a calm and collected manner. You finish the paper and then re-read through your answers, making any last minute corrections that are necessary.

The bell rings and you stop writing, the exam has finished. You feel positive and happy with your performance. You leave the room and feel confident that you have passed.

By going through this process your confidence will grow and negative thoughts and feelings of anxiety about the exam will start to recede.

Walking a fine line

The caveat to building your self-confidence is to not become over-confident. Confidence is unquestionably a good thing but being over-confident can adversely affect your exam performance.

Some medical students have quite literally never failed an exam when they arrive at Medical School. They feel indestructible and can't even imagine failing. This is unlikely to still be the case by the time that they have finished Medical School. The bad news is that nearly everyone reading this book will fail an exam at some point during their medical career.

If you become overly confident, the risk is that you will 'take your foot off the gas' and stop studying or study too little. Even the most confident student will fail if they haven't absorbed the necessary knowledge. Even when your confidence is high, keep chipping away and stick to study plan to avoid an unpleasant surprise on results day.

Key points to remember:

- ✓ Intelligence isn't the only predictor of academic achievement
- ✓ Self-confidence is also an excellent predictor of exam success
- ✓ Concentrating on positive thoughts will improve confidence
- ✓ Visualization is a great way to develop a positive attitude towards exams
- ✓ Being over-confident can adversely affect your exam performance

The Importance of a Good Nights Sleep

"There is a time for many words, and there is also a time for sleep."
Homer, The Odyssey

Pulling an 'all-nighter'

On several occasions over the years I have decided to 'pull an all-nighter' and stay up to study for an exam the following day. On some occasions it was because of a lack of preparedness or anxiety, sometimes it was due to peer pressure with flat mates doing the same, but on every occasion it was both unnecessary and counterproductive.

During my years working as a junior doctor, sleep became a luxury and I experienced great difficulty balancing my work commitments, social life, hobbies and exam preparation. I often got by on 5 hours of sleep or less but started to notice that my ability to learn and my performance were suffering as a consequence.

Studies by the Division of Sleep Medicine at Harvard Medical School have shown that the short-term gains from sleeping less are heavily outweighed by the detrimental effects of sleep deprivation. Most people require between 7 to 9 hours of sleep to be sufficiently rested and perform to the best of their potential.

Why do we need sleep to learn?

The cognitive effects of sleep deprivation are far reaching and it is known to adversely affect brain function in a number of different ways. A variety of different studies have linked sleep deprivation with irritability, mood changes, impaired judgment, increased stress, decreased creativity and even with symptoms of attention deficit hyperactivity disorder.

It has long been recognized that sleep and memory are closely interlinked. Memory formation has been shown to be both enhanced and stabilized by sleep. Different phases of the sleep cycle are associated with different types of memory formation, but Rapid Eye Movement (REM) sleep that occurs in the later stages of the sleep cycle, usually between 6 and 8 hours, is very important for people that are currently attempting to learn new facts. During the REM stage of sleep the brain is processing the previous day, removing unnecessary details and consolidating new knowledge that has been learned. If you sleep too little, not enough time will be spent in REM sleep and the learning process will suffer as a consequence.

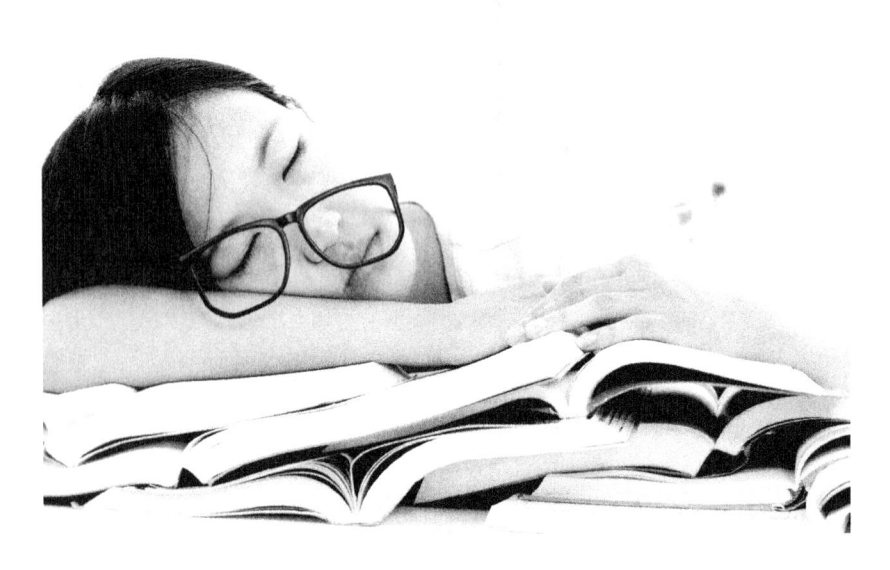

It is well recognised that sleep and memory formation are closely interlinked.

In addition to this, recent work by the Sleep and Neurophysiology Laboratory at the University of Rochester, has shown that sleep has an even more vital function. This research showed that there are numerous toxins released by the central nervous system as a consequence of the neural activity that occurs whilst awake. These toxins are processed and removed from the brain whilst we are asleep. If these toxins are not removed it is thought that it can impair our higher functioning and learning capabilities. Furthermore, it has been postulated that sleep deprivation may increase the risk of neurological diseases such as Alzheimer's disease, as a consequence of a build up of these toxins.

What else does sleep deprivation do?

In addition to the adverse effects on cognitive function, sleep deprivation has also been shown to have an association with a wide variety of serious health conditions. People that sleep more have longer, healthier lives.

Cortisol levels rise when the body has had inadequate sleep, resulting in central fat deposition and a weakened immune system. Testosterone levels have been shown to fall in men, resulting in reduced libido and fertility. Carbohydrate metabolism and appetite are also affected and there is an increased incidence of obesity in individuals that have inadequate sleep. Sleep deprivation has also been linked with an increased risk of heart disease, stroke and type 2 diabetes mellitus.

Another very serious point worth noting is that lack of sleep is associated with impaired reaction times and a higher risk of accidents. A survey from the UK Royal College of Physicians in 2006 showed that junior doctors were at increased risk of motor vehicle accidents whilst driving to and from work, and that the most risky timing was when returning home from a night shift. Changes to shift patterns were instituted following this survey, to attempt to address this problem.

Dealing with night shifts

I have experienced disturbed sleep patterns and difficulty sleeping during many stages of my life. Shift patterns and working on-call as a junior doctor certainly contributed to this. On many occasions when working prolonged runs of night shifts my body clock became so confused that I had difficulty sleeping more that two or three hours at a stretch. This also corresponded with the period in my life when I was most active academically and sat a number of important postgraduate exams.

The irregularity of working night shifts and doing on-calls often caused me to feel exhausted at work and then be unable to sleep during the day. Trying to re-organize my sleep pattern following nights became a crucially important part of my exam preparation and I learned many important lessons about 'sleep hygiene' along the way. Sleep hygiene is a set of different practices that help to promote good quality sleep and daytime alertness.

Improving sleep hygiene

One of the best ways to ensure adequate sleep whilst on night shifts is to eliminate all noise and light from your sleep environment. I had blackout window blinds fitted in my bedroom and would also wear earplugs and a sleep mask.

Melatonin controls our sleep-wake cycle, with the pineal gland starting to produce it in the evening and levels peaking in the middle of the night. Blue light exposure in the morning then suppresses production and levels remain low until the evening, when blue light levels fall and it becomes dark again. Watching TV or reading from a backlit iPad in the morning when returning home from a night shift will suppress melatonin production and disrupt your sleep pattern further, so try to avoid this if at all possible. An alternative is to wear blue-light blocking glasses in the last hour or two before you go to bed. Better still, try listening to an audiobook or some gentle music before you go to bed.

It is very tempting to load up with caffeine when working night shifts. This will certainly give you a boost when working on your shift but caffeine can stay in your system for between 6 and 10 hours. I stopped drinking coffee altogether on night shifts, and it definitely improved my sleep pattern, but if you feel that you must have a cup try to do it in the first hour or two of your shift only.

Try to also avoid drinking alcohol before you go to sleep. It will certainly make you sleepy initially but it will reduce your sleep quality and can shorten the period that you sleep for. You are also more likely to feel groggy and be less productive when you do wake up.

It has been shown that people that exercise have better quality sleep and trying to do some gentle exercise during your night shifts can help facilitate improved sleep. The caveat is that strenuous exercise too close to bedtime can cause increased alertness and delay falling asleep. Try to go for a walk or a gentle jog or swim before your shift to see if this helps your sleep when you return home after the shift but avoid exercising when you get home and are preparing for bed.

When all else fails, try to grab a nap whenever you can. If your shift is quiet try to take it in turns to get a short sleep whilst at work. If you work in a team try to organize a short sleep break for each member and cover for each other in turns. If it becomes busy or an emergency crops up it is very easy to be woken up, and you will almost certainly be fresher and more alert to deal with the situation.

Key points to remember:

- ✓ A good night's sleep is more important than all-night studying
- ✓ Sleep deprivation impairs memory formation and cognition

- ✓ Sleep deprivation is also associated with a wide variety of serious health conditions
- ✓ Junior doctors' work patterns can disrupt sleep patterns severely
- ✓ Take measures to improve your 'sleep hygiene' to improve your sleep quality

Food For Thought

"Your diet is a bank account. Good food choices are good investments." Bethenny Frankel

You are what you eat

Diet is often neglected by medical students and doctors, especially in the run up to exams. It is all too easy to eat an unhealthy diet during the revision period, binging on quick and easy snacks and junk food to save time and drinking energy drinks as a 'quick fix' for waning energy levels.

Not only is this terribly unhealthy, there is also compelling evidence that eating unhealthily can impair your exam performance.

There is a well-known saying that 'you are what you eat' and this is very true. To be fit, healthy and perform to the highest of your capabilities requires a balanced and healthy diet, and it is very important not to overlook this during your exam preparation.

Stay hydrated

Water is the most vital part of any healthy diet, it is a major constituent of our bodies and makes up about 60 to 65% of an adult human's body weight. Water has numerous vital functions and is needed for cellular maintenance, neurotransmission, transport of nutrients, metabolic reactions, body temperature regulation and waste elimination. An average healthy individual should drink between 1.2 and 1.5 litres of water per day, and these requirements increase in hot weather and with exercise.

Doctors are notoriously poor at remaining well hydrated, and one slightly tongue in cheek study published in the 2010 Christmas BMJ highlighted this. A case-control study was designed to compare urine output between junior doctors working in an intensive care unit with the patients for whom they were responsible. The study showed that 22% of doctors were classed as being oliguric and being 'at risk' of acute kidney injury, and that the doctors were more likely to be oliguric than their patients. Clearly, we as a profession need to be better at managing our own hydration status.

One study published in the European Journal of Clinical Nutrition in 2003 showed that dehydration is a reliable predictor of impaired cognitive status. Another study, published in the Journal of Nutrition in 2012, showed that mild dehydration caused headaches, increased perception of task difficulty, reduced concentration and low mood. It is not difficult to see how these effects could easily compromise both your study and exam performance.

Aim to drink 1.2 to 1.5 litres throughout the day and increase this figure if you exercise. Keep a bottle of water at your desk and snack on fruits with a high water content such as melon, peaches, pineapple and oranges. It is also important not to wait until you are thirsty to drink because thirst is a sign that you are already dehydrated. Try to avoid drinking sugary carbonated drinks and too many caffeinated drinks as these tend to have a diuretic effect and will dehydrate you further.

Eat healthy fats

Fats have received a lot of bad press over the years but the tide is slowly turning and there has been a gradual realization that fats are an essential part of our diet.

The human brain is made up of almost 60 percent fat and most of this lies within cell membranes. In fact, essential fatty acids (EFAs) are among the most important molecules that determine the brain's integrity and ability to perform. Fatty acids also provide the brain with a valuable energy source and are important for the maintenance of serotonin and dopamine levels. Furthermore, EFAs are not synthesized within the body and can only be obtained from dietary sources, so it especially important to make sure that your diet contains an adequate supply.

The best fats to consume to optimize brain function are omega-3 fatty acids. These appear to be particularly important for cognitive function and their use has been researched as a potential treatment for a variety of neurological conditions including Alzheimer's disease, depression and attention deficit hyperactivity disorder.

There are three types of omega-3 fatty acids: alpha-linolenic acid (ALA), eicosapentaenoic acid (EPA) and docosahexaenoic acid (DHA). Of these, it is the DHA that is most abundantly found within the brain and that appears to be most important for cognition. DHA is mostly found in marine sources, so try to make sure your diet contains plenty of oily fish such as salmon, sardines and herring. If you don't like to eat fish then consider buying some omega-3 or fish oil supplements that are rich in DHA.

Not all fats are healthy and you should try to avoid a diet heavy in saturated fats and trans fats. These 'bad' fats displace the healthy omega-3 fatty acids and reduce the flexibility of the cell membranes within the brain. These stiff membranes limit the structural changes that are essential for cellular communication and may actually impair cognitive ability. Trans fats can also accumulate in synapses and impair neurotransmission. Make a conscious effort to eliminate fried foods, French fries and fatty junk foods from your diet in the run up to your exams.

Eat 'superfoods'

The term 'superfoods' has been used a great deal over recent years within the diet and fitness industry. Although there is clearly no quick fix substitute for a healthy, balanced diet, there are a number of foods that have been claimed to have a positive effect on cognition and brain function.

Many nutritionists believe that if you are only going to add one 'superfood' to your diet that it should be blueberries. It is claimed that they have a wide range of positive health effects including having a protective effect against heart disease and cancer. Blueberries are packed full of vitamins A, C and E and also contains high concentrations of antioxidants including flavonoids and acanthocyanins. Blueberry flavonoids are thought to increase cerebral blood flow and interact with signal pathways that are important for brain cell survival. Their ingestion has been linked to improvements in cognition, such as improved attention span, memory enhancement and increased learning ability. Animal studies have also shown that blueberries may have a role as a potential treatment for dementia and Alzheimer's disease.

Eating foods that are high in vitamin C is also a good idea in the run up to your exams. Bell peppers, leafy green vegetables like kale, kiwi fruits and berries are all examples of foods that have a very high vitamin C content. Vitamin C is essential for the development and maintenance of healthy cerebral blood vessels and is also necessary for creating neurotransmitters such as dopamine. It is also a potent antioxidant that helps lessen oxidative stress to the body. Several studies have suggested that vitamin C has a protective effect against cognitive impairment and more research is currently underway looking at vitamin C supplementation for cognitive health.

Evidence is also accumulating that vitamin K helps to improve cognitive function. It is thought that vitamin K plays an important role in maintaining the white matter region of the brain by supporting myelin sheaths, protecting axons and facilitating the speed at which the brain functions. One particular study undertaken at the University of Montreal in 2011 showed that a diet low in vitamin K resulted in significant cognitive deficits in rats when compared with a group of rats that had a high vitamin K diet. Foods that have a high vitamin K content include kale, spinach and broccoli.

Eat nuts and seeds

Nuts and seeds are rich in many nutrients that have a variety of beneficial effects, and recent research has suggested possible benefits for cognitive performance.

Walnuts, which bear an uncanny resemblance to the human brain, may also improve brain function. Walnuts have a high omega-3 fatty acid content and are also rich in vitamin E, vitamin B6 and anti-oxidants. One study looking at the effects of a walnut rich diet in rats showed that it improved memory and cognitive performance.

Flax seeds are another healthy 'brain food' that is rich omega-3 fatty acids. Flax seed oil contains high concentrations of alpha-linolenic acid, which is used by the body to produce both EPA and DHA. They are not as good a source of DHA as fish oils but they provide an excellent alternative for people averse to eating fish.

Another nut to consider eating as a healthy revision snack is the cashew nut. Cashews are an excellent source of magnesium, which has been shown to increase cerebral blood flow. Almonds have also been cited as having potential cognitive benefits due to their high phenylalanine content. Phenylalanine converts to tyrosine, which acts as a precursor to the production of several neurotransmitters, including dopamine. It has been postulated that eating foods rich in phenylalanine may result in increased mental acuity.

Drink coffee and eat dark chocolate

Caffeine, also known as trimethylxanthine, is the world's most commonly used stimulant, with 80% of Americans estimated to use it on any given day. The most well known source of caffeine is the bean of the *Coffea Arabica* plant, which is used to make my favourite beverage, coffee. Coffee has been used in human society for hundreds of years and is reported as being discovered in Ethiopa in 800 A.D. Caffeine is also present in other drinks such as tea and numerous soft drinks and energy drinks.

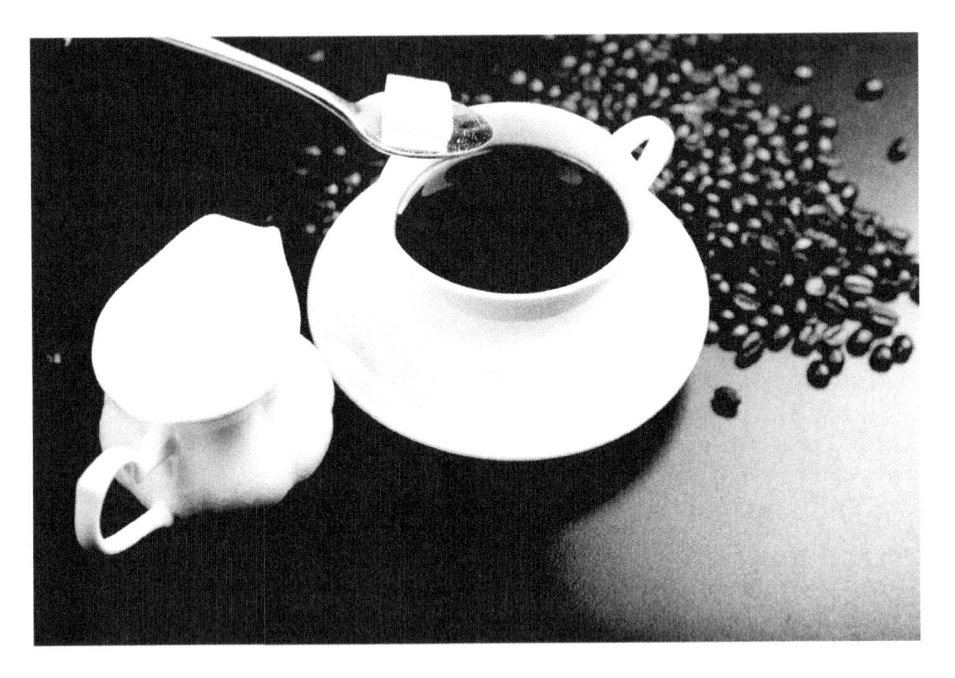

Caffeine ingestion can improve attention span and concentration at lower doses.

Caffeine is a stimulant that has a diverse range of effects on the central nervous system, including improved attention span and concentration at lower doses. It has also been shown to reduce mistakes caused by drowsiness in shift workers and improve performance during sleep deprivation. The effects start within an hour of ingestion and last for between 5 and 8 hours. Starting your day's revision with a cup of coffee will help to focus you for the task at hand and another cup with lunch may help to get you through the afternoon energy slump. I usually also drink a cup of coffee an hour or so before any exams that I sit.

It is worth noting that coffee and other sources of caffeine should be ingested in moderation. Caffeine also has some negative effects, particularly if taken in large quantities. If you drink too many cups of coffee you should expect to experience jitteriness and mild anxiety-type symptoms. It can also cause sleep disturbance and is an addictive substance with a recognized withdrawal syndrome.

Dark chocolate has powerful antioxidant properties and also contains caffeine. In addition to caffeine it also contains other stimulants such as theobromine and phenylethylamine. Theobromine has similar effects to caffeine but its stimulant effects are less pronounced. Phenylethylamine has a similar biochemical structure to amphetamines and causes release of dopamine and endorphins. A couple of squares of dark chocolate is a great way to enhance your focus and concentration whilst treating yourself to a delicious snack at the same time.

Key points to remember:

- ✓ Avoid snacking on junk food during your revision period
- ✓ Drink plenty of water and stay well hydrated
- ✓ The best fats to consume to optimize brain function are omega-3 fatty acids
- ✓ Eat plenty of 'superfoods' and snack on nuts and seeds
- ✓ Drinking coffee in moderation can improve attention span and concentration
- ✓ Treat yourself to some dark chocolate as a brain-boosting snack

Healthy Body, Healthy Mind

"True enjoyment comes from activity of the mind and exercise of the body; the two are ever united." Wilhelm von Humbodlt

The value of exercise

I have already mentioned how I have used exercise to help me with my exam preparation at several points throughout this book. Many people stop exercising before important exams as they perceive that they simply no longer have time for it.

I strongly believe that exercise is one of the most fundamentally important things that you can do whilst preparing for exams. Not only is exercise an excellent way to relieve stress and anxiety, it also has powerful neurophysiological effects that are advantageous for learning and memory.

Healthy body, healthy mind

Exercise increases cerebral blood flow and makes oxygen and vital nutrients more available to the brain. This increase in circulation also enhances energy production and waste removal. Exercise also causes the release of epinephrine from the adrenal glands, which has a stimulant effect and increases awareness and the ability to concentrate.

Numerous different studies have demonstrated a relationship between exercise and improved cognitive function. Aerobic exercise has been shown to promote neurogenesis and increase grey matter volume and increase neuronal activity. These changes have been associated with improved cognitive function and improved mood.

We know that the chronic stress of exams and studying increases cortisol levels in students. Having excess cortisol levels interferes with neurotransmitter function and has been shown to impair memory. Another valuable benefit of exercise is that, when done regularly, it increases the threshold for cortisol release. This makes the body more able to the cope with the effects of stress and less likely to suffer the detrimental effects of cortisol upon memory whilst studying.

Short bursts of moderate- to high-intensity exercise have been shown to induce a large increase in phenylacetic acid levels. Phenylacetic acid is the primary metabolite of phenylethylamine, the same stimulant that is present in dark chocolate. The euphoric effects that many people experience after exercising has been attributed to this and it also has the effect of increasing focus and concentration afterwards. For this reason, any studying done immediately after a short burst of high-intensity exercise can be particularly productive.

Exercise has also been shown to offset some of the effects of aging upon cognitive decline. One study that used MRI to measure brain volume in people over the age of 55 showed that individuals that had done the most exercise and were the fittest had the greatest brain volumes.

Consider exercising before your exam

There is also compelling evidence that a short burst of exercise before your exam can improve exam performance. Recent research by Dr. Charles Hillman at the University of Illinois showed that an acute bout of moderate exercise increased attention and academic performance in children.

Two groups of children were looked at: the first underwent a 20-minute period of aerobic exercise on a treadmill, and the second group sat and rested for 20 minutes. Both groups had event-related potentials (ERP) measured using electroncephalography (EEG). The children in the exercise group performed better in an academic achievement test and also showed increased ERP activity.

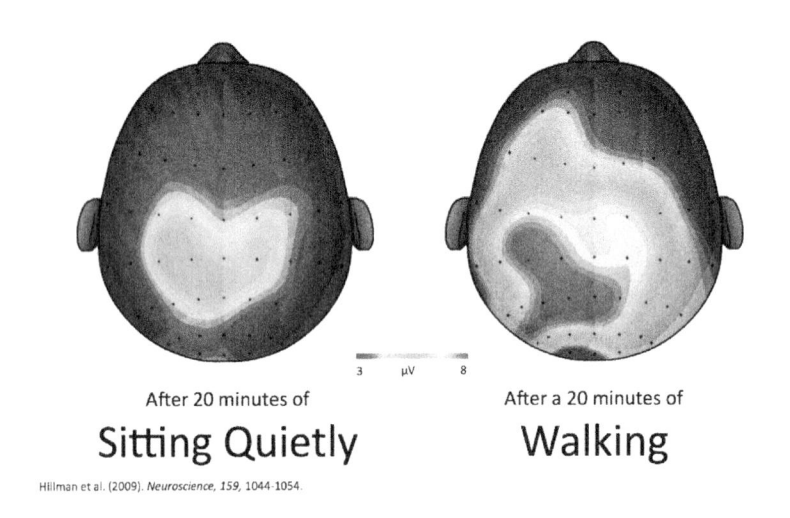

After 20 minutes of
Sitting Quietly

After a 20 minutes of
Walking

Hillman et al. (2009). *Neuroscience, 159*, 1044-1054.

Image of ERP activity provided courtesy of Dr. Charles Hillman, University of Illinois

Of course it does not necessarily follow that these results will be the same in adults but it is certainly worth considering taking some exercise the morning before your exam, or at least walk to the exam instead of driving or catching the bus.

Key points to remember:

- ✓ Exercise is a great way of relieving exam stress and anxiety
- ✓ Studies have demonstrated a relationship between exercise and improved cognitive function
- ✓ Exercise helps to offset the effects of chronic stress induced cortisol release
- ✓ A short burst of exercise before your exam may improve your performance

Meditation and Mindfulness

"Meditation can help us embrace our worries, our fear, our anger; and that is very healing. We let our own natural capacity of healing do the work." Thich Nhat Hanh

What are meditation and mindfulness?

Meditation, in its basic sense, is a way of releasing our minds and 'decluttering' our brains from day-to-day thoughts. It can help us filter out seemingly important sensory inputs and focus on our more spiritual beings. Meditation has been practiced in a variety of different forms for thousands of years. Meditation is referenced in the Hindu Vedas, some of which were written before 1000 BCE.

Mindfulness is when we become deliberately aware of the present, without judging the situation. It is a way of living consciously, with the goal of making healthy choices that impact our entire lives and those around us. The term 'mindfulness' is derived from the Pali-term *'sati'*, which is an essential part of Buddhist practice.

Although these meditative practices have their origins in Eastern religions they don't need to be based on any specific belief systems. They have increased dramatically in popularity over the past decade or so and today many people practice regularly.

Meditation and mindfulness are now commonly employed in modern psychology to alleviate a variety of conditions including depression and anxiety.

How can they help with studying?

There is now a large body of research that suggests that meditation and mindfulness can help to relieve stress and anxiety. They can provide an excellent means for relieving exam induced stress and gathering your thoughts during your study period. It is not known exactly how meditation works to combat stress but it has been postulated that it has effects upon the sympathetic nervous system.

The value goes deeper than just stress relief though, and there is also now evidence to show that students that practice mindfulness can enhance memory capacity and improve academic performance. A recent study from the Department of Psychological and Brain Sciences at the University of California showed that 2 weeks of mindfulness training improved test scores on a reading-comprehension test and working memory capacity. It also reduced the occurrence of distracting thoughts during the test.

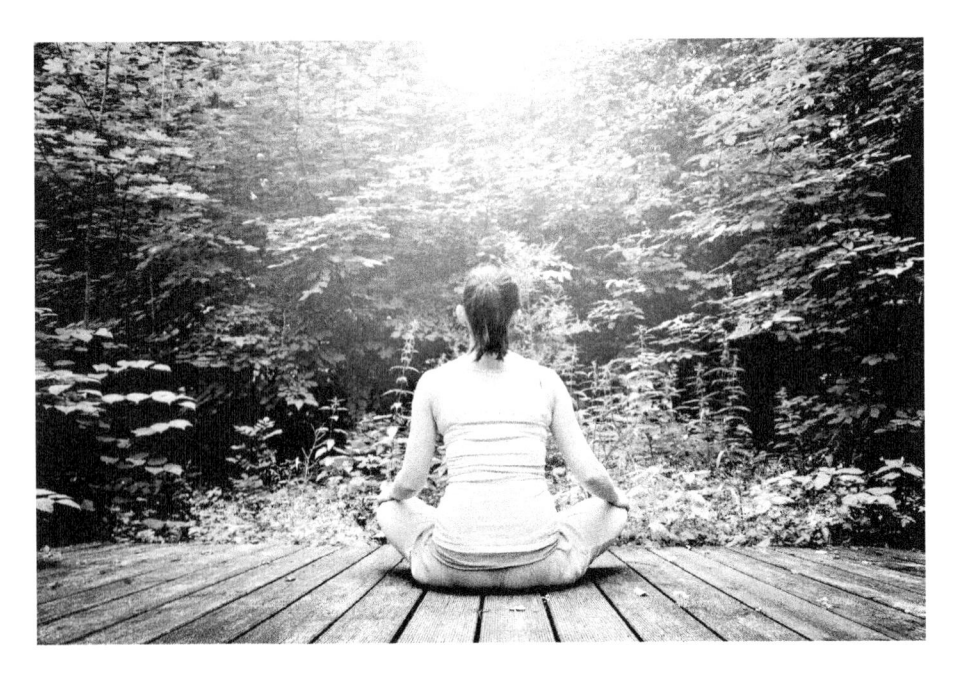

Meditation can help to relieve stress and anxiety and also increase memory capacity.

How to meditate

For the uninitiated it can be very difficult to sit for long periods and have an 'empty mind'. There are many guided meditation courses available where a teacher will help you to understand the process and get started. For myself, I found that starting with just a few minutes and then building up slowly to a longer duration helped me to adjust to the process. Try to practice, even if just for 5 or 10 minutes initially, on a daily basis so that it becomes a habit. Many people can quickly achieve 30 minutes or an hour of meditation in this manner. There are also many books and audiotapes available that can guide you through the process.

One way to meditate is to focus and concentrate on one particular thing. This could be as simple as focusing just on your breathing or perhaps thinking about a single word or staring at the flame of a candle. Find a quiet, dark, calming environment, as free from distractions as possible. Most people sit cross-legged, but if you find this uncomfortable to start with you could sit on a chair or even lie on a bed. Every time your mind wanders, let the thought go and then try to re-focus your concentration again. This particular type of meditation is very good for improving your ability to concentrate.

Mindfulness meditation should be approached in a slightly different way. Again, find a calm, quiet setting but this time try to observe any wandering thoughts that drift into your mind. You should not try to engage with these thoughts or judge them but rather be aware of them and try to ascertain how they make you feel.

There are numerous other ways to meditate, and yoga and tai chi practice can also have similar benefits. Some people have a preference for one particular type of practice whilst others practice a combination.

If you would like to learn more about meditation and mindfulness, the Oxford Mindfulness Centre is an excellent resource: http://www.oxfordmindfulness.org

Key points to remember:

- ✓ Meditation and mindfulness have a wide range of benefits and can help to relieve exam stress and anxiety
- ✓ Mindfulness can also enhance memory capacity and improve academic performance
- ✓ Start with short periods of meditation and build up gradually to longer durations

PART 5

FINAL PREPARATION

The Last Few Days

"When you are in any contest, you should work as if there were – to the very last minute – a chance to lose it. This is battle, this is politics, this is anything." Dwight D. Eisenhower

It is never too late

The final few days before your exam are vitally important. You will be tired, your nerves will be at their worst of any stage and it can be very easy to lose focus and direction with your study. It can seem overwhelming at this stage and it can sometimes feel as if there is too little time to learn anything of value.

Despite there being little time left there is still a great deal that can be achieved and these last few days might actually be the most important stage of your preparation.

Return to the syllabus

When there is about a week remaining it is a good idea to return to the syllabus again. By this stage you should be very familiar with its content and have an intimate understanding of what is required by you to pass the exam.

Earlier on in this book I suggested dividing the major topics within the syllabus into three 'traffic light' groups:

- Green - Topics that you have a good understanding of;

- Amber - Topics that you are familiar with but require more work;
- Red - Topics that are unfamiliar to you and are likely to require the most work

By this stage the contents of these three groups will have changed from when you first assessed the syllabus. The red 'traffic light' group should now be much smaller than the others. These are the priority areas that you should now spend your time focusing on. Review your notes on these topics and make flashcards on them, concentrating on the key points that are vital to achieve a good understanding.

The amber 'traffic light' group is your next priority. If time allows, practice some sample questions focusing on these areas to make sure that you have solidified your knowledge. In the last week little or no time should be spent looking at topics within the green 'traffic light' group.

Looking at the syllabus now should also boost your confidence. Looking at the large areas that are now marked green will allow you to see how far you have come and how much you now know.

Schedule a final study group meeting

At this stage it can be very easy to shut yourself off from the outside world and become isolated. Try to schedule in a final meeting with your study group to ensure that this doesn't happen. Arrange it so that each person in the group brings something personal to the agenda. If there are any topics or concepts that your are struggling with at this stage, the easiest and least time consuming way of gaining an understanding is to have it explained to you by someone who grasps it well.

Use your flashcards

By the final week before the exam I have usually created a database of flashcards, each containing key facts about important topics. A great way to break up your study is to give these cards to someone else and get them to test you on them. The person testing you doesn't need to have an intimate understanding of the subject matter as the cards will guide them and allow them to correct you on knowledge gaps. Ask a friend or a flat mate to test you when you are too tired to read or sit practice questions. My long-suffering wife has spent many hours fulfilling this role patiently over the years and it has helped me tremendously.

Making the most of your short term memory

Memory degrades very rapidly and psychologists estimate that we forget half of information presented to us within one hour and 70% within 24 hours. That being said, a great deal of information can still be committed to your short-term memory within the last 24 hours before the exam.

Really focus in on areas that you have had difficulty with in this time period. You may not be able to remember any of these last minute facts a week from now but as long as you can recall them in the exam tomorrow that won't matter. Using some of the memory tricks outlined earlier in this book, such as creating mnemonics and the mind palace principle, can aid your memory retention further and increase the amount of information you can commit to your short-term memory.

The last day

Try to get up early and start your revision as soon as possible on the final day before the exam. Consider doing a last minute mock exam or some question practice at some point during the day as a 'test run' for tomorrow.

Don't work too late into the day and leave yourself some time to relax and unwind in the evening. Go to bed early and get a good night's sleep, safe in the knowledge that the hard work has been done now and you are ready for the task that lies ahead tomorrow.

The last few days 'do's and don'ts'

Do:

- ✓ Return to the syllabus and focus on areas in the red 'traffic light' group
- ✓ Organize one final study group meeting
- ✓ Use your flashcards to help fill knowledge gaps
- ✓ Use mnemonics and the mid palace principle to maximize your short-term memory

Don't:

- ✗ Give up in the final stages and lose focus
- ✗ Shut yourself off from the outside world and become isolated
- ✗ Stay up late studying on the final night before the exam

Re-sits

"It's fine to celebrate success but it is more important to heed the lessons of failure." Bill Gates

Getting over the failure

Failing any exam is a difficult experience, particularly for medics, who are so accustomed to academic success. People experience a wide range of emotions following the failure of an exam. Some feel embarrassed, others feel angry and some become depressed. Many people lose confidence and direction after exam failure and it can be difficult to come to terms with starting the process again.

The chances are that you dedicated many months of study preparing for the exam and made numerous sacrifices in your personal life. Postgraduate medical exams can also be expensive, as are many of the courses and books that people use to prepare for them.

One of the best ways of dealing with the failure in the early stages is to talk to your family, friends and tutors. You will quickly discover that they are not disappointed in you and you will probably be surprised to discover how many of them have been through a similar experience. Online forums are another place to seek solace and advice from others that have failed the same exam. Failing an exam is not the end of the world, although it may seem that way initially. The fact of the matter is that you will almost certainly get another chance to sit the exam. Nearly every doctor has failed an exam at some point in their career, and some of the very best clinicians I know have had tremendous difficulty passing exams.

It is very important to take some time off following the exam and to not throw yourself straight back into revising. The process of preparing the first time will have been exhausting and you will need to re-charge your batteries before starting again. Make sure that you spend some time doing some of things that you sacrificed whilst revising or perhaps even take a short holiday. Slowly but surely the initial disappointment and upset of failure will subside and you will feel ready to let go the initial failure and start again.

Finding the positives

There is no way to undo the failure of an exam but there are actually many benefits moving forwards. You will undoubtedly have a far greater knowledge of the required subjects than when you first started your revision process, and all of the work that you have already done will help you tremendously with your preparation for the re-sit. You will also have notes and flashcards that you can use again and an intimate understanding of the syllabus.

Having actually gone through the experience of sitting the exam the first time around will have produced a familiarity that will help to calm your nerves when the time for the re-sit comes around. Think of your first attempt as a 'trial run' for this attempt, which you ARE going to pass.

It may seem difficult to accept to begin with, but find these positives and allow them to help you; the experience will make you a much stronger candidate the second time around.

Don't make the same mistakes again

About 18 months after I qualified as a doctor I attempted the MRCP Part 1, a notoriously difficult exam with a high failure rate. I went on to fail this exam, but by a relatively small percentage. Looking back I lacked confidence and self-belief and hadn't prepared properly as a consequence.

When talking to a friend that had passed the exam at the same sitting I realised that he had approached his preparation in an entirely different way to me. Not only had he dedicated more time to study, he had been more organized, spent more time doing practice questions and used a different textbook that was more focused on the needs of that particular exam.

I had clearly made several mistakes in my preparation process the first time around. When preparing the second time around I paid careful attention to the advice of my friend and the adjustments that I made helped me to clear the exam easily on the next attempt. This experience also helped me greatly with my preparation for the exams I have sat subsequently.

Talk to friends and colleagues that have sat the exam and try to work out what they did differently. Be honest with yourself about the mistakes that you made the first time around and allow this to help you make adjustments for this attempt.

Don't give up

One sure way to never pass an exam is to give up and not try again. Determination and willpower will get you through the re-sit and allow you to achieve your goals. It is very important not to be afraid to try again.

There are many examples of highly successful people that have failed initially but then managed to turn around their fortunes because they didn't give up.

Louis Pasteur was considered to be a mediocre student as an undergraduate and his physiology Professor told him that his 'theory of germs is ridiculous fiction'. He failed his first attempt at his *baccalauréat scientifique* exam in 1841 but managed to pass it at his second attempt the following year. Louis Pasteur went on to make numerous astonishing scientific discoveries. His 'ridiculous theory of germs' and his subsequent discoveries of the principles of vaccination, microbial fermentation and pasteurization have saved countless lives since then. He is now considered to be the father of modern microbiology and one of the finest medical minds from history.

Another very famous example of someone that did not give up despite initial failure is Thomas Edison. He was told by his teachers that he was 'too stupid to learn anything', he was also fired from his first two jobs for being 'non-productive'. It is alleged that it took Edison 1,000 attempts to successfully invent the electric light bulb, and when asked by a reporter 'how does it feel to fail 1,000 times?' He replied 'I didn't fail 1,000 times, the light bulb was an invention with 1,000 steps'.

Re-sits 'do's and don'ts'

Do:

- ✓ Talk to your family, friends and tutors to help you deal with the failure
- ✓ Take some time off before you start preparing for the re-sit
- ✓ Try to find the positives and allow them to make you a stronger candidate for your re-sit

Don't:

- X Feel embarrassed about your initial failure
- X Make the same mistakes you made the first time around again
- X Give up!

On The Day

"Your mind will answer most questions if you learn to relax and wait for the answer." William S. Burroughs

The big day has finally arrived!

After many months of hard study, the day of the exam has finally arrived. Hopefully you had an early night last night, slept well and have awoken refreshed and ready for the big day. If you didn't sleep well don't panic, as your sympathetic nervous system will kick in shortly and get you through the day.

Grab a decent breakfast that isn't too heavy. Avoid sugar-laden cereals that will cause a 'sugar crash' and a subsequent drop in energy levels. A meal containing protein, for example some eggs, or something like porridge, that will release energy slowly throughout the morning is ideal. I usually also have a cup of black coffee with my breakfast before an exam because of its mild stimulant and cognitive enhancing effects.

Having put in so much hard work, which has given you the best possible chance of passing, make sure that you get to the exam on time. Get there at least 15 minutes before the start of the exam and ideally aim to be there half an hour before so that you have extra time in case of traffic problems or unforeseen delays. If you are late you will have less time to complete the questions and under some circumstances you might not even be allowed to sit the exam. Getting there early will also allow you some time to focus yourself, relax and mentally prepare yourself for the task at hand.

If you can, try to fit in some gentle exercise before the exam, perhaps a brisk stroll or a light jog, as this has been shown to have cognitive benefits and improve exam performance.

Make sure that you have everything you need

Pack your bag the night before so that you are not in a rush on the day of the exam. There will probably be a checklist provided by the exam board; pay careful attention to this list so that you have everything you need. You will almost certainly need at least one form of photo identification and your exam admittance letter or ticket.

Think about taking spare pencils, pens and erasers. It is a good idea to have a watch or desk clock so that you can carefully monitor the time remaining in the exam. I would also recommend having a decent sized bottle of water with you so that you can maintain optimal hydration throughout the exam, if you are allowed to take drinks in with you.

Make sure that you haven't got anything with you that is forbidden. Most exams forbid the use of mobile phones and other electronic devices. I can't think of any exam that allows you to take in textbooks or notes. Being found having forbidden devices or materials will lead to you being dismissed from the exam and result in an automatic fail.

It is very important to be comfortable in the exam room and you should dress accordingly. Dress in layers so that you can add a layer if you feel cold or take off a layer if you are too warm. If you are sitting an OSCE or a viva make sure that you carefully adhere to the dress code and are suitably presented.

During the exam

At the start of the exam the steward will usually give you a series of verbal instructions. Listen carefully to what they have say as you may need this information during the exam. You will be told about the exam regulations and policies and also other important information about how to take toilet breaks, what to do if you need assistance and whether you will be able to leave early if you have finished.

When the exam starts read the instructions very carefully before looking at the questions or entering a station. Marks are frequently lost by nervous or over-confident candidates that have overlooked key information at the start of an exam. I can recall whilst sitting my mock A-levels as a schoolboy answering too many questions from one section of the exam and not enough from another. As a consequence of this very avoidable mistake I lost vital marks and didn't get the grade that I had hoped for. Fortunately it was a mock and not the real thing, and I have been careful not to repeat this error since.

Work out the timing of the exam carefully and divide your time between questions accordingly. If certain questions are worth more marks than others then allow more time for those questions. Also allow some time for reading through and checking your answers at the end of the exam.

If you are sitting a written exam, quickly look through the paper once before you start, to gain an overview of what is required of you. Then re-read each question more carefully in turn as you proceed through the exam. Make sure that you understand the question before you attempt to answer it, and underline any key information in the question text. Marks are easily lost by reading questions incorrectly, and again this is a very avoidable mistake. If you are writing essays or short answer questions ensure that your writing is neat and legible. If your answers are the highest possible quality in terms of content, but unreadable due to sloppy handwriting, you are not going to score many marks. If you know that your handwriting is difficult to read and this has been an issue for you in the past, consider printing your text.

Have a plan for your strategy in the exam before you go in. By now you should have sat several mock exams and have a good idea about what works best for you. Some people like to methodically work through an exam whilst others like to start with questions about the topics they know best, in order to get off to a good start. Whatever method you choose don't spend too much time dwelling on questions that you are unsure about; instead, mark the question, move on and return to it after finishing the questions you can answer well.

Dealing with problems during the exam

One of the biggest fears of candidates is that their mind will 'go blank' during the exam. If this happens take a deep breath and relax, return to the question and re-read it. This will allow you to regain your focus and will often trigger your memory and allow you to answer the question. If it doesn't, simply move on to the next question and return to this one at a later stage. The chances are that by the time you return to it you will be calmer and able to recall the information required.

If you think that there is a problem with a question or a mistake in the paper put your hand up and notify one of the stewards. This way the exams officers can be informed of any potential problems and this can be taken into account during the marking of the exam. They will also be able to give you guidance as to how to answer that question and they may choose to make an announcement to all of the candidates to ensure that no one is disadvantaged. Don't dwell on this, and continue with your exam as normal as soon as this has been dealt with.

Another common problem encountered in written exams is hand cramps or pain. This can be extremely annoying and is often a problem in essay papers that require a lot of text. It is often caused by gripping the pen too tightly or pressing down too hard on the paper. Make sure that you have a pen with a large, comfortable grip and hold it as gently as you can. Try to write using your arm and not just the hand and wrist. The reality is that even with great writing technique, a good pen and a loose, relaxed grip you will almost certainly get some hand or elbow discomfort in a lengthy essay based examination. When the inevitable happens, put the pen down and rest for a moment. Try shaking your hand out and stretching your wrist and fingers, and hopefully this will alleviate the discomfort and allow you to return to writing.

If you find that you are running out of time, don't panic. Realising that this is the case is the most important thing. Take a moment to look at the remaining questions in the paper and check how much time you have left. Split the remaining time proportionately between the remaining questions. Try to be as economical as possible with your answers from this point forwards.

After the exam

Relax and take it easy now, the exam is finished and nothing more can be done at this stage. It is entirely natural to want to discuss the paper with your friends but try to avoid an in-depth 'post mortem' of the paper.

Go home, relax and try not to think about the exam too much until the results are published. You should take comfort in the fact that you have prepared well and given yourself the best possible chance of passing as a consequence.

On the day 'do's and don'ts'

Do:

- ✓ Make sure that you get to the exam on time
- ✓ Make sure that you have everything you need
- ✓ Read the exam instructions and questions carefully
- ✓ Take comfort in the fact that you have prepared well

Don't:

- ✗ Eat a sugar-laden breakfast and suffer a ' sugar crash'
- ✗ Waste time dwelling on questions you can't answer
- ✗ Perform an exam 'post-mortem' with friends after the exam

Closing Thoughts

"Being deeply learned and skilled, being well trained and using well-spoken words: this is good luck." Buddha

As I look back over my life in medicine over the past 20 years or so I am overwhelmed by the wide range of rich experiences that I have been fortunate to have been exposed to. I have changed tremendously as an individual and I had no idea that the road would have led me to where I am now. I have had many happy moments and many deeply sad moments, I have been witness to both miraculous events and awful tragedies, sometimes in the same day.

Medicine is a career pathway that will challenge you throughout your working life and the exams that you face along the way are only one small part of the adversity that you will go through. On many occasions I have questioned the value of some of these exams and wondered if they were unnecessarily difficult. I can now see that this is not the case and that sitting the exams was a crucial part of my development as a doctor. My successes and failures contributed equally and taught me many important life lessons. They are not just about the accumulation of facts and knowledge but represent so much more. Passing your medical exams will unlock the door to your future as a doctor and will help to forge you into an individual that will help many, many people over the course of your life.

I hope that the content of this book helps you to face this particular part of your own personal journey and that you can learn from my own experiences of sitting exams. I also hope that by reading this book you can avoid making some of the mistakes that I made along the way and that the journey is a little easier as a consequence.

Try your best, don't give up and have faith in your own abilities.

Good luck and I sincerely hope that you pass!

Dr Marc Barton

About the Author

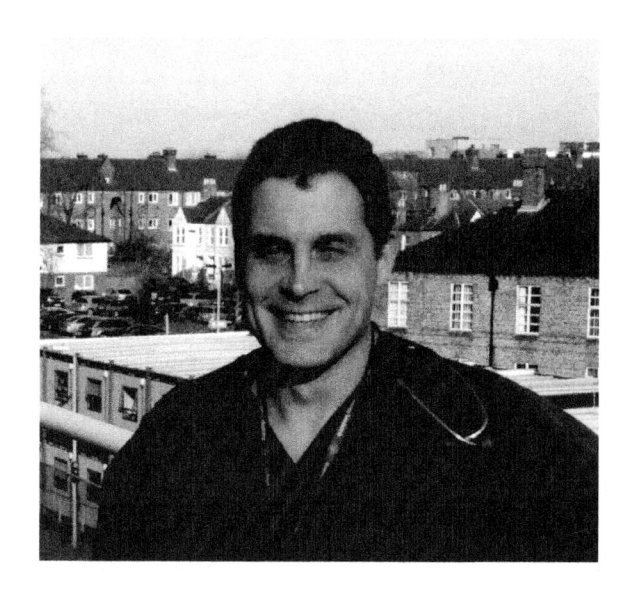

Dr. Marc Barton qualified from Imperial College School of Medicine in 2001. Since that time he has worked in a variety of different medical specialities. He worked as a GP partner from 2006 until 2008 and more recently as a higher specialist trainee in Emergency Medicine.

He has gained a formidable reputation as an exam candidate and in addition to passing a Bachelor of Science degree and Medical Finals as an undergraduate, he has also passed three postgraduate membership exams and two postgraduate diploma exams. He has an active interest in medical education and a wealth of experience teaching both medical students and doctors.

In his private life he is a devoted husband and father of three children. He is also a lifelong martial artist and regularly teaches Jiu Jitsu in his spare time.

Printed in Great Britain
by Amazon